W9-CEW-119

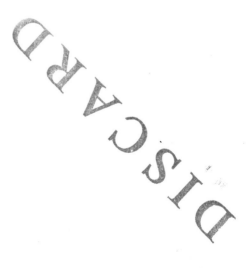

The Organ Shortage Crisis in America

THE ORGAN SHORTAGE CRISIS IN AMERICA

Incentives, Civic Duty, and Closing the Gap

Andrew Michael Flescher

GEORGETOWN UNIVERSITY PRESS / WASHINGTON, DC

The publisher is not responsible for third-party websites or their content. URL links were active at time of publication.

Library of Congress Cataloging-in-Publication Data

Names: Flescher, Andrew Michael, 1969- author.
Title: The organ shortage crisis in America : incentives, civic duty, and closing the gap / Andrew Michael Flescher.
Description: Washington, DC : Georgetown University Press, 2018. | Includes bibliographical references and index.
Identifiers: LCCN 2017025225 (print) | LCCN 2017026296 (ebook) | ISBN 9781626165441 (paperback) | ISBN 9781626165434 (hardcover) | ISBN 9781626165458 (ebook)
Subjects: LCSH: Donation of organs, tissues, etc.—United States. | Donation of organs, tissues, etc.—Moral and ethical aspects.
Classification: LCC RD129.5 (ebook) | LCC RD129.5 .F58 2018 (print) | DDC 362.17/830973—dc23
LC record available at https://lccn.loc.gov/2017025225

♾ This book is printed on acid-free paper meeting the requirements of the American National Standard for Permanence in Paper for Printed Library Materials.

19 18   9 8 7 6 5 4 3 2 First printing

Printed in the United States of America

Cover design by Martyn Schmoll. Cover image by Shutterstock.

CONTENTS

ACKNOWLEDGMENTS

For seven years I have served as the medical ethicist on our hospital's Organ Donor Council, the last three of which as a living donor advocate. A living donor advocate, the presence of which is required by federal regulation whenever a transplant occurs, certifies that every individual poised to donate an organ understands what is about to take place, is aware of the risks involved, has given full and informed consent, knows what the next weeks and months of life will look like and how to take care of himself or herself after surgery, and is aware of the medical center's grievance process should concerns arise at any point in the process. As the first point of contact for living donors, the living donor advocate serves as an unconditional and independent resource. In the time I have spent protecting the interests and health of donors, they have, in turn, taught me something about what it means to be a courageous and flourishing human being. It is our job to look out for them; it is their self-assigned calling to look out for a dying family member, friend, or stranger.

Giving a part of one's body to another who is in desperate straits is never in the medical interests of the donor. Yet, in talking to donors I have been given the near-singular impression that donating an organ is a fulfilling and inspirational activity. Donors consistently describe the decision as a "no-brainer" and one to which they refer with an unwavering buoyancy and determination. Increasingly I have come to wonder what informs such confidence and, more pointedly, why, given this confidence, there are not more donors. This book is the fruit of an investigation into answering this question, an inquiry I might not have undertaken if ten years earlier I hadn't spent hours with my uncle during a few of his visits to the facility in Toronto where he received dialysis. I owe my uncle for helping me understand and sympathize with someone in kidney failure who lives beholden to strictly scheduled dialysis appointments. These sessions define the limitations around which such an individual must organize and live the entirety of his or her life.

My exposure to this reality, which profoundly shaped my professional identity in the years after, is, therefore, in a sense an accident. This said, 10 percent of the population worldwide is affected by chronic kidney disease, and kidney disease remains the ninth leading cause of death in the United States. What makes these particular figures so interesting is that, unlike the numbers associated with other serious health ailments from which patients suffer and die, we have the medical technology at our disposal to be able to do something about kidney disease. How to recruit living donors in an ethical *and* efficient manner, however, remains a subject of vigorous debate, given both the large number of individuals on the waiting list and the new possibilities that contemporary technology has made available. I have spent the bulk of my career asking questions about what motivates human beings to act with compassion, and this work reflects the culmination of my moral, intellectual, and personal preoccupations.

I have been fortunate to think about and discuss these issues with brilliant and diverse colleagues at Stony Brook University and Stony Brook Hospital. I want to thank Steve Knapik, Carrie Lindower, David Harris, Amanda Fortuna, and Dawn Francisquini, among the many who have served with me on the Stony Brook Hospital Organ Donor Council, for making available to me the indispensably eye-opening experiences that made a project like this more than an abstraction. Steve Knapik, Stony Brook Hospital's living donor coordinator, in particular deserves my gratitude. He made sure the most interesting cases came across my desk and arranged to have me scrub in at Stony Brook's operating room in order to witness firsthand a laparoscopic nephrectomy, followed by a kidney transplantation in the adjacent operating room. Steve, along with Carrie Lindower, then the administrative director of Stony Brook's Kidney Transplant Program, secured me a prominent voice at the annual national conference for transplant professionals (NATCO). Without this clinical exposure to the transplantation process, and to the clinicians involved in the process, I would not have been able to write this book.

I thank my incredible colleagues in the Program in Public Health at Stony Brook University. At various stages of this project Lisa Benzscott, Sean Clouston, Norman Edelman, David Graham, Lauren Hale, Amy Hammock, Evonne Kaplan-Liss, Rachel Kidman, Jaymie Meliker, Catherine Messina, Tia Palermo, John Rizzo, Jamie Romeiser, Carrie Shandra, and Dylan Smith gave me the tools I needed to interpret the data, just as they pressed me to be as precise as possible in reporting it. As the lone humanist in the Program in Public Health, I am the beneficiary of their more-than-a-layman's methodological acumen in the sciences and social sciences, which was crucial at several junctures in this book. I am grateful to them and to the two graduate students with whom I have worked, Candace Stewart and Brooke Nepo, for the indispensable feedback they all gave me over the last three years.

Thanks also to the organizers and attendees of conferences at which I presented: the Lloyd Erskine Sandiford Center and the Queen Elizabeth Hospital in Barbados (in May 2012) and the NATCO in Louisville, Kentucky (July 2015) and Orlando, Florida (July 2016). Finally, I am grateful to Peter Singer and colleagues at the Center for Human Values at Princeton University, who invited me to present much of this work to the DeCamp Bioethics Seminar just before it was scheduled to go to press. In particular I am grateful for the last-minute feedback from Eric Gregory, Liz Harman, Anne Barnhill, and their graduate students for their analytic insights and for presenting a couple of interesting objections to my arguments I had not yet considered. This work was made possible by virtue of all of these individuals and because of a sabbatical awarded to me by Stony Brook University's School of Medicine.

This is my third book with Georgetown University Press. An author could not be more fortunate to have an enduring relationship with a particular press. I am immensely appreciative of Richard Brown, director of the press, as well as his staff, for continuing to believe in me and in my work. This book is dedicated to the memories of my uncle, David Flescher, and his brother, my father, Robert Flescher.

Introduction:
The Organ Shortage Crisis in America

In the United States, nearly 120,000 individuals are in need of a healthy organ. Every ten minutes a new name is added to the organ transplant list, while on average twenty people die each day waiting for an organ to become available.[1] The shortage is especially disconcerting given that since organ transplantation became accepted as sound medical treatment, we have never had better technology—or so little occasion to avail ourselves of it. "It is the best of times and the worst of times," writes Dr. Amy Friedman, the medical director of LiveOnNY (New York's organ procurement organization), channeling Dickens. The frontiers of nephrectomy technology have advanced enough over the last fifteen years that today we have the ability to render dialysis medically defunct. The survival rate of a kidney that is donated from a cadaver graft is about 93 percent after one year, compared to over 97 percent in the case of living donors (89 percent and 95 percent, respectively, after three years). Recipients of kidneys usually go on to live normal lives following their operations. Sadly, however, too often they "wait with dignity for the life-saving organ that never comes."[2] Nephrectomy technology has so improved that, in principle, if not yet in practice, we have the means to all but eliminate the organ shortage problem, just as we have eliminated the blood shortage problem over the last fifty years. The distinction between what is possible and what is practical is important to note because the realization of such a dream hinges on a precious good—willing donors—without which the solution is purely academic.

Roughly 100,000 of the individuals awaiting an organ need a new, functioning kidney. This is significant because, other than a lobe of the liver, the kidney is the only transplantable organ one can donate while still alive.[3] In a telling editorial for the *New York Times* that appeared in early May 2014, psychiatrist and medical ethicist Sally Satel addressed an uncomfortable reality

1

pertaining to the growing shortage of organs: to fix the problem we can no longer rely on cadaveric donations. "We can't solve the issue merely by getting people to sign organ donor cards—though everyone should—or even by moving to an opt-out system, under which we would harvest people's organs at death unless they had earlier indicated they didn't wish to donate them. These solutions can only do so much, because relatively few people die in ways that leave their organs suitable for transplantation."[4]

Even if the United States were to become like the twenty-four "opt-out" countries in Europe for whom willingness to donate one's organs is assumed unless otherwise stated, we would still be far from closing the gap in this country between available organs and needy recipients.[5] The reason for this is a result of several things. Aided by new technologies, we are getting better at staving off brain death; seatbelts are being improved and cars are getting safer; more and more laws are meant to increase safety on the road, and these laws are becoming more enforceable; and we are able to keep people alive longer on dialysis. These and other factors combine to indicate that, over time, if we continue to rely primarily on a cadaveric donation program, in which only 1 percent of a population who die are able to donate their organs, the organ shortage gap will continue to widen.[6]

At the moment, living donors account for about one-third of all kidney transplants performed in the United States.[7] However, recently there has been a decline in the number of living donors as well as in the percentage of living donors relative to overall kidney donors.[8] This unfortunate statistic is in part responsible for a larger trend: since the late 1980s, the organ supply has increasingly failed to keep pace with demand.[9] Yet, at medical centers nationwide, the discussions among donor councils—such as the one on which I sit at Stony Brook Hospital in Stony Brook, New York—about how to improve organ donation rates almost invariably center around cadaveric donation. We spend hours discussing, for example, how to make the referral process more efficient in cases of brain death, how to craft statewide legislation so as to encourage more registration, and how to think creatively about expanding the criteria for eligible donors. Notwithstanding the important improvements to the referral system that these conversations spur, cadaveric donation itself as a means of recruiting donors has shown increasingly limited results year after year.

In response to this situation, some suggest that artificial, biomedically engineered organs are the answer for those whose natural organs are failing. At the present moment, however, this is not a solution. According to optimistic estimates, we are at least fifteen to twenty years away from perfecting such technology.[10] This again raises the question of living donation and, in turn, the challenge of motivating healthy young and middle-aged adults to give their kidneys to the loved ones or friends they know are in need and—if we are to make a maximal impact on the increasing shortage—to strangers as well. Hence the inquiry for discussion here: What is the most efficacious means of attracting prospective living kidney donors? Is it financial incentive? If so, of what sort? Or is it altruism? Could it be some combination of the two? Is it even possible for financial and altruistic incentives to be combined?

The question of which among these alternatives is better—and whether the alternatives stand in competition—remains untested because we as a society are generally uneducated about the difference living donors can make and the opportunities that exist for individuals to become living donors, should they desire to walk this road.[11] In response to the growing shortage, which has rightly come to be called a "crisis" by almost all OPOs (organ procurement organizations) across the country, it has become vogue among transplant surgeons and others to furnish novel and compelling arguments for legalizing the sale of organs in order to increase the available pool. But will the creation of a free and regulated market for organ trade increase a donor's motivation to "give the gift of life" (which, to be accurate, would no longer really be a gift)?

Traditionally, any objection to legalizing the sale of organs has been raised on the basis of one of three kinds of ethical misgiving: (1) the practice may lead to discriminatory and oppressive conditions for the impoverished; (2) the practice is tantamount to *commodification*, that is, the debasement of a good once it acquires a price tag; and (3) the practice is medically unsafe. Each of these objections is important and needs to be qualified carefully. But in theory each could be satisfactorily addressed, and today, in light of the exigency precipitated by the growing organ shortage problem, we have a reinvigorated motive to do so. The analysis here will review the merits and shortcomings of these objections and consider whether, when combined, they are enough to deter the libertarian or staunch capitalist from wanting to legalize the sale of organs.

A subsequent but important question quickly arises: Would legalizing the sale of organs, *aside* from the ethical misgivings just mentioned, achieve the pragmatic goal of recruiting enough informed and willing donors to reduce the shortage problem? And if we are to reject legalizing the sale of organs on the basis of skepticism about a policy's ability to reduce the shortage, what constructive proposal(s) might work in its place? Going somewhat against the grain, I will examine possible solutions to alleviating the organ shortage crisis apart from legalizing the sale of organs and explore incentives to becoming a living donor for the sake of fellowship and concern for others.

MOTIVATIONS FOR GIVING, ESPECIALLY OF PRECIOUS GOODS

In the 1970s it became illegal to sell blood in the United States. Yet over the last fifty years we have managed to get a handle on the blood supply shortage. This leads us to speculate whether it could be possible to address the organ shortage problem the way we have historically dealt with the blood supply. We regularly meet the needs of hemophiliacs, the victims of trauma, and so forth with voluntary donations procured through blood drives. However, unlike blood, bodily organs are not able to be replenished. Donating a kidney (or lobe of the liver) is a bigger deal than donating blood. In August 2014, in my capacity as a living donor advocate and a member of the organ donor council at Stony Brook, I spent a day observing two adjacent operating rooms where a mother donated a kidney to her son.

The first procedure, a nephrectomy, took about four hours, even though it occurred laparoscopically. During the first three hours the surgeon attended to the painstaking process of cutting through several layers of fat in order to reach the kidney that was to be removed. For the safest and most precise extraction in laparoscopic nephrectomies, the area around the kidney has to be "blown up" so the surgeon can maneuver without the obstruction of nearby organs or tissue. The process of cutting through these layers of fat and then isolating the kidney to be removed causes scarring and leaves the donor feeling considerably bloated and uncomfortable for two to four weeks following surgery. Dealing with the aftermath of surgery is not the only thing living donors must manage. For the rest of their lives they must carefully watch their sugar intake, they will never be able to take ibuprofen or other anti-inflammatory medications, and they risk renal failure should the remaining kidney be damaged in a sports-related or other contact injury.[12] There is no question: giving a kidney to another is a life-changing event for the donor.

Many advocates for organ donation believe it would therefore be foolish for someone to undergo a nephrectomy without adequate monetary compensation. When I first met her in 2012 following a conference in which we had debated whether kidneys should ever be for sale, Dr. Amy Friedman, a compassionate and prominent advocate for the cause of organ donation, told me she would be hesitant to give her kidney to someone she didn't know and that she certainly would not do so without being paid. She is a mother, she explained, and she could one day be pressed into service to donate to her child. This potential turn of events, combined with the known physical hardships, are enough for her to be reluctant to recommend that one altruistically give one's kidney to a stranger. While it might be deemed admirable to sacrifice for the sake of another, because of the costs involved she acknowledges no notion of some moral "ought" by which one could reasonably come to feel *compelled* to give one's organ to another. I mention all of this because one thing should never be lost for any proponent of living donation: despite recent technological advances, donating one's kidney represents a significant and costly toll to the donor, even in the vast majority of cases when the surgery goes as planned.[13]

Over the last ten years transplant surgeons like Friedman have joined forces with free market economists to craft, collectively, a vocal and passionate defense of the right and freedom one has to be able to do what one wishes with one's body, including profit from it when the self-sacrifice entails significant risk.[14] Since donating one's organ while still alive comes with formidable costs, they argue, we need an adequate inducement to compensate the donor. Mark Cherry, a libertarian and professor of applied ethics, argues for the permissibility of the creation of an organ market as a morally viable means for making human body parts available. He states that such a market is the most just and most efficient (available) means to procuring bodily organs and the means most compatible with the primary Western religious and philosophical value that one is the ultimate steward over one's own body.[15] To those who worry that putting a price tag on an organ might push away some who may be willing to donate without financial compensation, proponents press critics to make the case for the supposed contradiction they claim to notice between the motivation to help others and the pursuit of self-interest. The philosopher Janet Radcliffe Richards challenges the traditional prohibition against creating a market for the sale of organs using this logic:

> There is no necessary connection at all between payment and non-altruism or between non-payment and altruism. If a father who gives a kidney to save his daughter's life is acting altruistically, then so, by the same criterion, is one who sells his kidney to be able to pay to save his daughter's life. . . . So even

if there were any justification for holding as a principle that organ donation was unacceptable unless altruistic, it would still not support the prohibition of payment. In fact the only way to get from an altruistic premise to the required conclusion would be *defining* "altruistic" as "without payment." . . . The altruism requirement, in other words, looks suspiciously like a mere restatement of the non-selling requirement, with spurious moral knobs on.[16]

Richards reasons that the association between altruism and nonpayment is at best a nominal and arbitrary imposition on the part of the moralist to apply an additional definitional criterion to a notion that should merely require that the given good be authentically rendered. Money is no more than a currency, so why can't it be a currency that facilitates, rather than supplants, altruism?

It is a legitimate question. Why should human beings be thought of rigidly, *either* as selfishly motivated *or* as purely altruistic, and, furthermore, why should these states be thought to exist in competition with one another? Many people, as Cherry, Richards, and others rightly point out, make a financial living performing tasks that improve the lives of others in such a manner so as also to bring those individuals great enjoyment. Where service to others ends and replenishment of self begins is impossible to quantify neatly, and in any case why should there be a need for this quantification? The physician, the educator, the civil engineer, just to pick a few examples, save or enhance the lives of others and as a result get to reap both the financial rewards of their labor and receive the blessing of affecting the world for the better. This concurrency of objectives need not be restricted to the context of making a living. We might imagine a committed advocate for reproductive rights being financially compensated for her willingness to serve as a surrogate for a couple trying desperately to conceive or a stalwart member of a small community getting paid to donate his or her family's estate for the purpose of creating a village center from which everyone will benefit. That the lender of one's womb or donor of one's land is being compensated in these two examples does not necessarily diminish the giver's passion for the greater sake for which the gift is earmarked.

It seems rash to oppose, as a rule, altruism and self-interest. Facets of each frequently appear in the other. To concede as much, however, is not to grant that the selling of one's organs to recipients in need is relevantly like the example of the surrogate or the landowner. One might accept the theoretical point that self-regard and selflessness are compatible motivational states yet still resist the additional contention that one can expect the performance of self-sacrificial acts on behalf of the other in need to go more smoothly upon payment. While there may be no strict contradiction to the idea of overlapping motivations, it does seem to miss a critical psychological insight: a rendered good *can* mean something different—something more—to the giver when it is rendered free of compensation. It might be that offering cash for certain goods, or certain *valuable* goods, has the effect of changing those goods from what they used to be prior to the transaction.

This is an admittedly counterintuitive claim to make. From the perspective of the one dying from a failing organ, a new organ uniquely serves as a lifesaving good. Any further qualification of this good, to paraphrase British philosopher Bernard Williams, is arguably "one qualification too many" from the perspective of the one whose life hangs in the balance. The spirit with which a kidney is offered is one thing; the kidney itself is another. And the latter saves the life. Such commonsensical reasoning reflects the perspective of the many who want to legalize the sale of organs. We are reminded of the sentiment popularized by Amy Friedman that it is high time to stop "waiting with dignity for the organ that never comes." We should grant that the saving of a life must be considered the highest priority, even if it could be established that paying for organs somehow cheapens the activity of procuring them. Nevertheless, in our process of setting priorities, we must still ask the critically important empirical question: Does the assigning of a price tag in fact positively impact the recruitment of willing donors?

It is the burden of the organ donor advocate who is worried about legalizing the sale of organs to demonstrate that givers of costly, valuable goods are not motivated by tangible incentives in the manner believed by proponents of creating a market for an organ trade. In endeavoring to assess this case, we must address the nature of what can be called "especially precious" goods. Especially precious goods are goods that are crucial, scarce, and nonreplenishable; by virtue of these three traits, especially precious goods transcend their tangible, material function. Bodily organs are one example species of the larger genus of especially precious goods. If we can determine something about what governs the exchange of bodily organs, we can also learn something about especially precious goods in general.

Our analysis of what governs the exchange of the especially precious good of a human kidney will be informed by my personal interviews of living donor individuals, most of whom did in fact end up fulfilling their initial intent to give a kidney to a recipient in need. Such individuals reported with passion and consistency that they wished not to be compensated financially for their gifts and, furthermore, that they would become upset upon learning it had become legal in this country to be paid for one's kidney after they were not paid.[17] These donors also reveal that they *do* have a "selfish" motivation to donate: namely, to connect with their recipient in some significant way.

It is interesting that upon giving the gift of life, donors wish not to remain anonymous. While the interviewed donors did not expect nor want to get paid, they almost always did want to get to know the organ recipient, and often not just in a superficial way; the donation was made in the context of a blossoming acquaintanceship that could strengthen into a real friendship over time.[18] Typically it was important to the donor that his or her gift be acknowledged, not for credit or reward but for the purpose of forging inroads into the "gift of life" community. This indicates that organ donation is a *social* activity.

Communal inclusion is its own powerful motivator, which is perhaps not so surprising if we examine countries in which donating one's blood or organs is more the norm than it is here in the United States. In Sweden, blood donors are sent automatic text messages when their blood has actually been used, thanking them for the difference they made in the life of another.[19] In Israel, registering to become an organ donor means higher placement on the recipient list simply by the simple fact of registering. These kinds of practices reflect values-based decision-making on the part of a citizenry and its leadership to participate in the promotion of a shared social good. In the United States, "celebration of life" banquets for the purpose of bringing organ donors and recipients together are becoming annually anticipated events during the month of April, national organ donor month. These events celebrate the connection between individuals in ever widening communities; the same basis for them would not exist if donors were merely contractually linked to their recipients. Such inspiring examples of "donation for life" communities that are forged by family, friends, and strangers coming together for a common cause raise the question of whether, with more public education, a living donation program could engender sufficient civic engagement to stem the tide of the growing shortage crisis in available organs.

A fairly well-known example will help shed some light. On July 22, 2003, Zell Kravinsky, a self-made millionaire who had already given away $45 million to various charities while saving money in the bank only for his children's future college education, snuck out of his house without his wife's knowledge and had his kidney removed in Philadelphia at Albert Einstein Medical Center, donating it to a complete stranger, a thirty-year-old African American woman named Donnell Reid. Prior to receiving Kravinsky's gift, Reid had to take a bus to and from her dialysis infusions every other day. When questioned by journalist Jason Fagone about what motivated his gesture of kindness (judged heroic or insane, depending on who you asked), Kravinsky's own reply is illuminating. Knowing something about dialysis, Kravinsky said he couldn't allow a person to endure it any longer if an action of his could prevent it. Reports Fagone: "Three hundred thousand-plus souls languish in dialysis—a blood-cleaning process that leaves you dog-tired and drained, six hours a day, three times a week. Zell decided he could spare part of himself to save a fellow human from this hell."[20] In response to those who asked about his motives, Kravinsky reverses the attention back on the questioner: How can we, in good faith, allow someone to languish if we can do something about it? Kravinsky's attitude toward giving reveals a sense of our shared civic duty. Even if costly, we ought to sacrifice for another if we can.

This unbending sense of self-obligation underscores a final point of inquiry: the theoretical emphasis on the tension that exists between the two kinds of incentive. Kravinsky's motivation can reasonably be described as "selfish" only in the sense that for him to be himself—for him to be *for* himself—his identity must be bound up with replenishing others. *This* sense of self (and self-interest) is incompatible with the motivational desire to attend only to, or even primarily to, one's own interests. Furthermore, saving a life is not the only important thing at stake when an organ is exchanged. When it comes to especially precious goods, the relational connection developed, communal solidarity, and social justice also hang in the balance. In fact, these "extra" goods are *part* of the good of the bodily organ. The situation is also not less complicated by virtue of the fact that we live in a capitalistic society and that we are accustomed to paying for things we want at the moment we want them (and, once paid, having those things as ours to enjoy without having to apologize for or explain our enjoyment). But this presumption has limits under exigent circumstances, such as when those things are rare and dear.

Capitalism does a poor job of fully explaining the psychological realities attendant to our giving nature. Some people are not motivated by money. Exceptional as he is, countless people like Zell Kravinsky exist, and many more would exist were their giving natures given a better chance to be triggered and then nurtured. Kravinsky is assuredly no more likely to donate because of the reward he expects to receive. Are altruistic donors like Kravinsky an anomaly, or are they individuals we can admire from afar but also emulate up close?[21]

While Kravinsky himself gave out of a morally demanding sense of personal obligation, he believed, like Gandhi, that this standard of civic duty should apply not just to himself but to everyone.[22] His inspiring example suggests the power of the incentive of civic duty, which remains undetermined from individual to individual. There is no reason to think that under the right circumstances it could not rival the incentive of being paid.

CIVIC DUTY

It would be hasty, and perhaps glib, to rush too quickly to pronouncements that "civic duty" means we must put ourselves in harm's way. One of the most characteristically revealing aspects of the sense of obligation felt by organ donors, and by those who make great sacrifices for others in general, is what such individuals report about their own actions—namely, that it is a personal compulsion that emanates from within.[23] They do not see their loving sacrifice as an obligation that strikes them as something they must do because of an external or foreign sanction. Civic duty will hardly serve, and should not serve, as a rival to financial incentive for recruiting willing donors if one is coerced into becoming involved in the hardship of others. The alternative to a paid service is a freely offered gift. A freely offered gift is rendered of one's own accord.

Civic duty, in the sense meant here, connotes not a top-down "ought" from the outside but community building and inclusion that emanates from within. The "duty" is really a reminder that we do not exist by ourselves in the world and we are always dependent on and needed by others. If one sees oneself as fundamentally alone—an individual unit who fends for oneself—then the notion of civic duty as an impetus meant to compel action will not be persuasive. For this reason it is futile to tell someone that he or she has a duty to care about someone else without first giving that person a way of seeing, understanding, and subsequently caring about the experiences of the person in need. When friends or acquaintances ask me why they should register as organ donors, reciting statistics about numbers of individuals on waiting lists isn't enough. Instead, I encourage them to spend a session with someone on dialysis: to witness the infusions, to listen to the person's description of what life is like when one is required on a regular basis to be sedentary for extended periods of time, to learn what it is to gain and lose substantial amounts of water weight week after week and experience painful muscle cramps as a result, and to hear about how hard it is to become employed or develop a career under these conditions. It is a movement of perspective-taking to consider the plight of one whose object of life is to survive rather than live.[24]

By spending time with people who are struggling, our connection to them deepens. This experience increases the likelihood that we will come to care genuinely about them and, in turn, desire to help them. Civic duty, in other words, is established not only, and not even mostly, by the cogency of a rational argument; rather, it is by the more natural transformations attendant to how we psychologically form attachments. Reasoning can get us to a place where we incur the cognitive burden to be receptive to the plight of others, but it is sympathy and fellowship that does the work of connecting. To put the point in another way: civic duty is recipient-oriented more than it is donor-oriented. One will be inspired to step into harm's way to benefit another not only because of the influence of moral or religious tradition, but also because one has spent time with a person in need and as a result has decided voluntarily to become involved. The recipient's voice, experience, and point of view represent powerful and active aspects of the giving process.

In light of this observation, it may be useful to contrast the scenario of egg or sperm donation, which occurs under conditions of anonymity and for which donors do (legally) get paid, as compared to the not-anonymous activity of organ donation, for which donors do not and cannot get paid.[25] If one of the principal ambitions of organ donation is to make it possible for donors to get to know recipients, what accounts for the difference between the two? The answer has everything to do with the ultimate purpose for which the giving act is undertaken. In the case of egg and sperm donation, the sacrifice is somewhat minimal, there is an undetermined period of time that elapses between donating and receiving, and a certain distance is assumed between the transacting parties. The process of egg and sperm donation is itself typically bureaucratic and consistent with the functional nature of the goods being exchanged—that is, as a strict means to an end. Regardless of whether human eggs or sperm *should* be regarded as "especially precious" for religious reasons or otherwise, our society does not treat them as though they are. The price tag for them assures the contractual nature of their exchange.

In the case of organ donation, on the other hand, anonymity would undermine the social relation affirmed by the proposed exchange. As sociologist Kieran Healy notes in the case of cadaveric donation, families of donors are almost without exception preoccupied with the recipient(s) of their departed loved ones' gifts.[26] They imagine an "idealized recipient, often resembling the loved one they may have lost."[27] As presented in the research of ethnographer Courtney Bender, even in instances of altruistic anonymous giving, such as cooking meals for people with AIDS, "the reproduction of social solidarity through generosity, obligation, and repayment [is] accomplished through gifts circulating among specific, known individuals."[28] Social solidarity fuels the gift exchange.

The notion of a gift is in this respect contingent on an expected relationship. According to Healy, this goes to the very definition of "gift." Invoking the anthropological insights of Marcel Mauss and Bronislaw Malinowski, Healy notes:

> A gift is something much more general than a present wrapped up and given on a special occasion. Rather, gift exchange can involve "any object or service, utilitarian or superfluous. . . . 'Gift' does not identify either the object or the service itself, or the forms and ceremonies of giving and getting. Instead, what makes a gift is the relationship within which the transaction occurs." In gift exchange, transactions are *obligatory*, the goods exchanged are unique or *inalienable*, and the exchange partners are *related* in some way beyond the specific transaction. Contrast this with the typical market relationship. In the market, exchanges are voluntary or formally free (no one is forced to buy or sell), the goods exchanged are fungible, and exchange partners are linked only by the contract governing that particular transaction.[29]

More than a gift is offered in gift-giving. As Healy puts it, gifts are not expendable; they are inalienable and they carry the mark of the giver with them wherever they go. Most goods, depending on the context, can be manifested either as gifts or as fungible, or tradable, items. In the case where goods have a relational component, however, they can only be exchanged as gifts—that is, as more than simply tangible items. When this relational aspect occurs, neither the identity of the giver or the recipient, nor the relationship between them, can be unlinked from the gift itself.

This is not to say that gifts are never misconstrued as fungible goods. From time to time valuable goods are not treated with the proper regard they deserve. Something that ought to have been ascribed with unique or inalienable status is considered something less. When this happens, a social cost is borne by future givers and receivers of this good. In the example of bodily organs, the cost pertains to the buy-in on the part of the general public to the raison d'être of organ or blood donation and other forms of other-regarding sacrifice.

A WORD ABOUT THE AUDIENCE AND PURPOSE OF THIS BOOK

This book is different than others I have written, wherein I assumed more distance from my subject. As before, I hope to educate my reader in a scholarly way about "the other," in this case the potential organ recipient. But here I harbor ambitions of an activism that, at some rhetorical risk, will have the effect of personally confronting the reader by virtue of asking some grounding questions about the nature of who we are as human beings and what motivates us.

I have hypothesized that when it comes to giving particular sorts of goods, market incentives do not afford a giver the same motivational push or internal satisfaction he or she gets when giving from a sense of social cohesion. Some research provides tentative support for such a claim. In one study conducted by Bruno Frey, the number of Swiss citizens who were contacted by the government about their willingness to live in (safely distant) proximity to a nuclear waste facility declined precipitously when they were offered money for their sacrifice.[30] (Initially, slightly more than 50 percent were prepared to have the waste facility nearby; when respondents were told that the Swiss government was offering substantial monetary compensation, the consent rate dropped to under 25 percent).

Frey's study gives credence to Richard Titmuss's controversial contention, articulated in his seminal book, *The Gift Relationship*, that an offer of financial reward "crowds out" other more powerful incentives, such as the desire to help others in need.[31] Titmuss compared blood donation rates for the years 1946 to 1968 in England and Wales, where the sale of blood was illegal, to those in the United States, where it was not. Counterintuitively, financial incentives squelched rather than supplemented the impulse to "help the fellow neighbor." One implication of Titmuss's crowding-out thesis is that we have the capacity to see ourselves in different ways: as relational individuals who do not count our assets relative to what others have going for them, or, alternatively, as negotiating individuals who vigilantly look out for number one. As the mantra goes, "once a commodity, always a commodity." But to say so is not to aver that all goods are commodities at the outset of their inception. We are variable in our identities relative to the other, and the goods we exchange are variable as well. It stands to reason that markets corrupt social relations by reducing interactions of exchange to a contractual experience.

We will take a close look at Frey's, Titmuss's, and others' studies involving different goods that indicate the incompatibility of these two relational states, between the self and the other. What are the merits of Titmuss's crowding-out thesis? Should it be accepted as is, or with modification? Is there a third alternative for solving the organ shortage crisis other than the capitalist's prescription of paying for organs or the purist's competing notion never to do so? We will explore possibilities for addressing the shortage once the lump-sum incentive is taken off the table and, looking beyond Titmuss, will introduce ways of seeing self-regard and self-sacrifice as ultimately compatible dispositions. For example, we will consider the advantages of paired exchanges (which involve four to six individuals; donors donate to other recipient[s] and in return their loved one receives a donation from an assigned matching donor); donor "chains" (which begin with one pure donor and end with one pure recipient but primarily contain donors willing to donate their organs on behalf of a loved one for whom they are not a match, as well as the recipients who are to receive one of these designated organs); systems that contain incentives for those who opt into a network; forms of financial compensation short of direct monetary payment; the importance of removing financial disincentives to donating; and the venues, such as "walls of heroes," that formally acknowledge donors' heroism. All of these innovations, when implemented somewhere in the world where there is an organ donor network, do not rely on lump-sum payment but nevertheless have in some way stemmed the tide of the organ shortage problem.

To date, a plausible proposal for how to confront the organ shortage crisis without legalizing the sale of organs has yet to appear in the literature of biomedical ethics or public health policy. Many volumes address the ethics of organ donation in general, such as Arthur Caplan's *The Ethics of Organ Transplants*, Nicholas L. Tilney's informal historical account of transplantation technology, *Transplant: From Myth to Reality*, Renée C. Fox and Judith P. Swazey's *Spare Parts: Organ Replacement in American Society*, and T. M. Wilkinson's *Ethics and the Acquisition of Organs*. These four books are historical in nature, covering ethical issues as wide ranging as religious resistance to and compatibility with the practice of transplantation, brain death definition and criteria, conflicts of interest between advocates for donors and recipients, expanding criteria of donor pools, and so forth. Other contributions to the field deal specifically with the blood and organ donor experience as it relates to altruistic motivation. Titmuss's classic, *The Gift Relationship*, was already mentioned. The social scientist Kieran Healy's *Last Best Gifts* seeks to test Titmuss's strong thesis—that offering financial compensation for blood, and presumably organs, "crowds out" more altruistic or civic-minded motives—through reference to several surveys that assess sacrificial motivation in society. Katrina A. Bramstedt and Rena Down's *The Organ Donor Experience: Good Samaritans and the Meaning of Altruism* provides a close reading of the testimony of organ donors, relying on anecdotal accounts of the motivation for "Good Samaritanship" in the context of organ donation. These three studies explore the power of altruistic giving in the context of self-sacrifice, but they do not necessarily provide a comprehensive theory of donor motivation. The volume of essays edited by Jason T. Siegel and Eusebio M. Alvaro, *Understanding Organ Donation: Applied Behavior Science Perspectives*, offers evidenced-based research conducted by sociologists and health psychologists seeking to establish the best means of testing and evaluating what factors contribute to donor motivation. The essays are methodologically technical; they address existing hospital, media, and university campaigns for the organ donor network and assess what such campaigns do effectively and ineffectively. Finally, a few books deal favorably with the rising wave of support among libertarians, transplant surgeons, and others for legalizing the sale of organs. Notable among these are *Kidney for Sale by Owner: Human Organs, Transplantation, and the Market* by Mark J. Cherry; *The Kidney Sellers: A Journey of Discovery in Iran* by Sigrid Fry-Revere; *Why Markets in Human Body Parts Are Morally Imperative* by James Stacey Taylor; and the most circumspect of them all, *Transplantation Ethics* by Robert Veatch and Lainie F. Ross (the latter also being a good general treatment of how to think more broadly about procurement).

All of these resources are useful and address a scholarly need in the expanding area of organ transplantation and medical ethics. This said, at present no work proposes a solution that both represents an alternative to legalizing the sale of organs and also proceeds from the assumption that altruism and self-interest might complement one another. The present work is written with the hope of addressing this opportunity by proposing some concrete solutions to the organ shortage problem that reflect the subtle and complex relationship between altruism and self-interest in instances in which especially precious goods are exchanged. It considers the most important ethical arguments both for and against legalizing the sale of organs, it delves into the phenomenon and implications of "commodification," and it suggests what a gift exchange powered by civic engagement might look like.

ORGANIZATION

Chapter 1 makes the strong case for the legalization of the sale of organs by introducing the disparate but related arguments for construing organs as commodities subject to acquiring value in the free market like any other item of value for sale. Chapter 2 considers the three objections to legalizing the sale of organs that have traditionally been raised by biomedical ethicists: (1) discrimination against the poor, (2) the commodification of a good based on its financial market value, and (3) unsafe outcomes. Each of these objections is serious, has more than one facet, and should give reflective ethicists pause even if one grants the notion that legalizing the sale of organs will automatically lead to an increase in the amount of available organs. While all these ideas have been discussed elsewhere, my way of synthesizing the ethical cases for and against legalizing the sale of organs has not appeared.

Chapter 3 begins from the supposition that the proponent of legalizing the sale of organs can go some distance toward answering the three ethical objections considered in chapter 2. I take seriously the proponent's concern about "waiting with dignity for the organ that never comes" and accept the utilitarian response that increasing the amount of organs, rather than giving for giving's sake, is what most ought to drive our assessment of whether or not to embrace a policy that calls for the legalization of the sale of organs. I then go on to argue that on these exclusively pragmatic grounds, legalizing the sale of organs will nevertheless not meet the goal of reducing the gap between available organs and organs in need. The case hinges on the notion that a private transaction of an especially precious good is never made between two parties only. Rather, precisely because of the preciousness of the good being exchanged, the exchange comes to assume a public character. This insight then builds to a comparison of the motivational efficacy of capitalistic incentives on the one hand and one's sense of civic duty on the other, especially in the case of critical, scarce, and nonreplenishable goods such as bodily organs.

That donors do have a strong interest in getting to know their recipients and their families suggests that altruism is not the polar opposite of self-interest. Based on testimony from donors poised to give the gift of life, chapter 4 explores the adage that "virtue is its own reward," especially in the case of a good that has both a tangible and an intangible component. Chapter 5 draws a picture of civic duty in action by applying this understanding of the relationship between altruism and self-regard to some recent but as of yet underdeveloped policies that rightly capture our attention due to their innovative nature. These include paired exchanges; donor chains; national policies enacted in order to give preference to those who opt into an organ donor network; incentives that provide compensation short of direct payment; and hallowed spaces that acknowledge the sacrifices of donors. The book concludes with a concrete suggestion—a modest first step—for how to begin to relieve the organ shortage crisis in America.

The case of organ donation, which involves both felt sacrifice and real benefits, underscores the importance of not "doing ethics" from an armchair. As we become more familiar with organ donation we will be less spooked by an appeal to our civic sensibilities. This is already happening in Europe and elsewhere. Of course, the best way to educate oneself is to spend time with a desperate potential recipient. He or she always serves as the reminder that altruistic donation is never just theoretical or symbolic.

Admittedly, the notion that we ought to become better acquainted with the plight of someone on dialysis for the sake of helping a stranger in need is a tall order. Steve Knapik, the indefatigable and compassionate living organ donor coordinator at Stony Brook Hospital, and many other living donor coordinators with whom I have discussed the matter are, like Amy Friedman, cynical about the prospect of donation in instances in which the donor and recipient do not know one another. While they would admire the person who stepped up to the plate to help someone previously unknown, these workers for the cause are reluctant to recommend that others go and do likewise. This is partly because they know that donating one's kidney means losing control over how it will be cared for by its new host. They are also aware of the possibility that at any time one could be called to donate to one's own family member, which is moot if one has already donated to a stranger. Finally, they are knowledgeable about the arduous nature of the surgery itself and its potential long-term consequences. They believe that while the desire to become a kidney donor is commendable, it is not something that should be associated with an "ought" in any binding sense, particularly in cases where donor and recipient are not kin.

These concerns challenge the thesis of this book: that living donation fueled by civic engagement represents not just a legitimate but perhaps the most viable solution to the organ shortage problem. My critic is understandably worried that from the start my project is fraught with an insurmountable idealism and naïveté. If seasoned and caring living transplant coordinators such as Knapik restrict what we mean by "standard" forms of living donation to mean only cases in which donors are family, then how optimistic can we be about expanding an anonymous living donation program?

My wager is that we should be considerably optimistic. Though we are not yet at a point where a nephrectomy is only minor surgery, we are still much closer to that than we are to being able to medically engineer organs.[32] When the "kidney donation as minor surgery" day does arrive, it will become plausible to imagine a world in which kidney "drives" are able to capture the public's attention in the way that blood drives do today. This book is penned with the expectation that ongoing innovation in medicine, combined with an increasing awareness on the part of healthy individuals of what it is like for someone to live with organ failure, will produce a society in which we come to expand what we mean when we "give the gift of life." More broadly, the discussion here is an investigation into what motivates people to give up precious resources for the sake of others on the occasions when they choose to do so. This investigation is undertaken in response to a current proposal to legalize the sale of organs, a proposal that assumes that the most powerful incentives are ones that appeal exclusively to individual self-interest. If I have been successful, I will have not only weighed in on a critical policy recommendation in the area of public health and medical care but will have also gone some distance in shedding light on what we humans are like when placed in the position to respond to others less fortunate.

NOTES

1. These statistics can be found at http://www.uwhealth.org/transplant/transplant-quality/10610, last accessed December 4, 2017. The Department of Health and Human Services updates these figures on a regular basis.

2. Dr. Friedman often mentions this phrase, or a version of it, in her writings and at conference presentations. See, for example, the transcript for the panel "We Should Legalize the Market for Human Organs," a debate among participants Lloyd Cohen, Amy Friedman, Sally Satel, James Childress, Francis Delmonico, and David Rothman, sponsored by the Rosencrantz Organization, at http://intelligencesquaredus.org/images/debates/past/transcripts/OrganMarkets-051308.pdf.

3. Six organs can be donated—namely, heart, lungs, full or partial liver, kidneys, pancreas, and intestines; tissue that can be donated consists of skin, corneas, bones,

tendons, veins, arteries, and heart valves. A cadaveric donor can save up to eight lives. Living donors can give only one kidney and a partial liver.

4. Sally Satel, "Why People Don't Donate Their Kidneys," *New York Times*, May 4, 2014, http://www.nytimes.com/2014/05/04/opinion/sunday/why-people-dont-donate -their-kidneys.html.

5. Technically speaking, the majority of these countries are not in the position to assume willingness to donate; they simply have a policy that permits the state to take cadaveric bodily organs unless one has opted out. Thus, willingness to donate is not, to be precise, assumed. According to surveys, about a fourth of the people would not agree to have their organs taken. The one exception is the country of Wales, which does presume consent. I thank one of Georgetown University Press's anonymous reviewers for pointing out this qualification.

6. Stephen J. Dubner, "Make Me a Full Match," *Freakonomics* podcast transcript, June 17, 2015, at http://freakonomics.com/radio/?radcat=radio-podcasts.

7. Annual data report from Organ Procurement and Transplantation Network (OPTN) and Scientific Registry of Transplant Recipients (SRTR), OPTN/SRTR 2012 (Rockville, MD: Department of Health and Human Services Health Resources and Services Administration, Healthcare Systems Bureau, Division of Transplantation, 2014).

8. J. R. Rodrigue, J. D. Schold, and D. A. Mandelbrot, "The Decline in Living Kidney Donation in the United States: Random Variation or Cause for Concern?," *Transplantation* 96 (2013): 767–73.

9. Kieran Healy, *Last Best Gifts: Altruism and the Market for Human Blood and Organs* (Chicago: University of Chicago Press, 2006), 24.

10. Despite recent press claims that we are just a few years away from 3D printing of usable organs, even charitable estimates on our ability to engineer viable bodily parts using this or other technologies predict success at least ten years into the future, and this is before we know whether the products such technologies yield will be able to function well in a living human body. While scientists have had some success artificially manufacturing skin, urine tubes, and blood vessels, as well as comparatively simple hollow or holding areas such as the bladder, we do not yet have the technology to create complex organs like kidneys, lungs, or a heart. Nor do we have any evidence that, once created, such organs will be able to survive for a reasonable amount of time in the body. The pioneer of biomedical engineering Gabor Forgacs recently estimated at the Select Biosciences Tissue Engineering and Bioprinting Conference in 2015 that we are still "several decades" from being able to biologically print or otherwise engineer a heart or liver. See Matt Davenport, "Print Your Heart Out," at http://cen .acs.org/articles/93/i10/Print-Heart.html, accessed June 22, 2017.

11. D. LaPointe Rudow et al., "Consensus Conference on Best Practices in Live Kidney Donation: Recommendations to Optimize Education, Access, and Care," *American Journal of Transplantation* 15 (2015): 914–22.

12. While the idea that biomedical engineering will significantly affect the organ shortage problem in coming years may be a fatuous notion, the idea that nephrectomies

will in subsequent years become easier for the donor to bear is not. Nevertheless, in small but meaningful ways the donor's life changes upon donation. Moreover, at present it is unknown the degree to which the removal of one of the two kidneys makes one susceptible later in life to type 2 diabetes, especially in cases where hypertension develops. This is therefore a cause for concern among living donor coordinators. Because assessing the precise cost of kidney donation is so hard to pin down, it is not as easy to make judgments about how feasible it will be to solve the organ shortage problem solely through campaigns of public awareness as it has been in the case of the blood shortage problem. For a discussion on the scant amount of information on the potential correlation between donating one's kidney and the subsequent risk of diabetes, see H. N. Ibrahim, A. Kukla, G. Cordner, R. Bailey, K. Gilliangham, and A. J. Matas, "Diabetes after Kidney Donation," *American Journal of Transplantation* 10 (2010): 331–37, http://onlinelibrary.wiley.com/doi/10.1111/j.1600-6143.2009.02944 .x/abstract;jsessionid=A05901C1EE76A6481BC3F092E024ADF1.f04t03. For a general discussion of complications following kidney donation (not just diabetes), see Neil Boudville and Amit X. Garg, "End-Stage Renal Disease in Living Kidney Donors," *Kidney International* 86, no. 1 (2014): 20–22, http://www.sciencedirect.com /science/article/pii/S0085253815302635?via%3Dihub.

13. At present the mortality rate for nephrectomies among living kidney donors is 3 in 10,000, which is, as far as major surgeries go, a very good statistic. The most well-known complications associated with the procedure, such as allergic reaction to anesthesia, pneumonia, blood clots in the lung, infection of the wound or urinary tract, and internal bleeding, are all rarer occurrences in nephrectomies associated with living donations than they are with other comparably invasive surgeries. This is because the population from which living donors come is among the healthiest in the United States.

14. A good example of a think tank that specifically takes on the cause of opening nontraditional goods to the open market is the Free Market Institute at Texas Christian University, which is increasingly catching the attention of organ procurement organizations across the United States. See on YouTube the second episode of the Free Market's series, *Free to Exchange*, specifically on the topic of legalizing the sale of organs: https://www.youtube.com/watch?v=dzZla4KSBPM&feature=youtu .be, accessed September 1, 2015.

15. Mark J. Cherry, *Kidney for Sale by Owner: Human Organs, Transplantation, and the Market* (Washington, DC: Georgetown University Press, 2005), 28–36.

16. Jean Radcliffe Richards, *The Ethics of Transplants: Why Careless Thought Costs Lives* (Oxford: Oxford University Press, 2012), 75–76.

17. This was the view of Lauren Muskauski, a hospital services specialist for LiveOnNY. Lauren donated her kidney to a stranger through a paired exchange. She stated in an interview that while she didn't expect and wouldn't have wanted financial compensation beyond a thousand dollars or so to help her defray the expenses of the donating process, if she were to learn that others were now legally allowed to get paid for donating a kidney, she would become angered by this development. Lauren created a blog in which she shares in engaging detail her journey toward donation.

See https://livinglegacymd.wordpress.com/2012/03/23/my-living-donation-journey-part-1-the-decision/.

18. Katrina A. Bramstedt and Rena Down, *The Organ Donor Experience: Good Samaritans and the Meaning of Altruism* (Lanham, MD: Rowman and Littlefield, 2011), 23, 145–46; and Kieran Healy, *Last Best Gifts: Altruism and the Market for Human Blood and Organs* (Chicago: University of Chicago Press, 2006), 116–17.

19. Jon Stone, "Blood Donors in Sweden Get a Text Message Whenever Their Blood Saves Someone's Life," *Independent*, June 10, 2015, http://www.independent.co.uk/news/world/europe/blood-donors-in-sweden-get-a-text-message-whenever-someone-is-helped-with-their-blood-10310101.html.

20. Jason Fagone, "What If Zell Kravinsky Isn't Crazy?," *Philadelphia*, May 15, 2006, http://www.phillymag.com/articles/what-if-zell-kravinsky-isnt-crazy/#XoUU2BdOp9TGU9JA.99.

21. About 3 percent of living donors are also "altruistic donors," or individuals who give a kidney or partial liver to a stranger. It is always possibly controversial when someone volunteers one's organ to one who is not a friend or family, and a responsible living donor advocate must make sure that the donor is fully informed, able to offer full consent, is mentally healthy, and not exhibiting some form of masochism or other unhealthy self-interest in offering his or her organ. Questions about Zell Kravinsky's state of mind captured ethicists' attention when he deceived his wife in order to donate his kidney to a stranger. Even beyond the question of Kravinsky's sanity, however, and assuming he did a wonderful thing for the sake of another, there remains the further distinction about whether he is worthy merely of our admiration or also our emulation. For more on the distinction between the admiration and emulation of moral heroes, see Flescher, *Heroes, Saints, and Ordinary Morality*, 5, 109–57.

22. See Fagone, "What if Zell Kravinsky Isn't Crazy?": "Donnell Reid, 30, [is] an African-American woman from Mount Airy who took the bus to her dialysis treatments every other day. They couldn't have been more unalike, but Zell still risked his life to save her from certain death. He goes as far as to call her his 'sister'—a sentiment worthy of Gandhi, Yitzhak Rabin and Martin Luther King, the 20th century's great martyrs to universalism."

23. Andrew Flescher, *Heroes, Saints, and Ordinary Morality* (Washington, DC: Georgetown University Press, 2003), 138–41.

24. In May 2012 I was invited to Barbados for a weeklong conference sponsored by Queen Elizabeth Hospital to explore the prospect of transitioning the country from a system of addressing end-stage renal failure, which relied exclusively on dialysis, to one that would begin to permit kidney transplantations. After appearing on television and radio programs touting the virtues of the new approach, the most memorable part of the conference culminated with a session in front of the country's health minister in which the country's first recipient of a new kidney exclaimed, "Before receiving this gift my goal each day had been to preserve my life; overnight it became again to live."

25. Sperm and egg donors in general have no wish to be invited into the community or share in the plight of reproductively challenged individuals pursuing

parenthood. It is quite the opposite. This was revealed a few years ago when legislation was proposed in countries across Europe to begin to keep confidential records of sperm donors so that children who wanted to know the identity of their biological fathers would have the ability one day to be made aware of this information. (Initially, these changes were proposed in response to ethical concerns about donors fathering many more children than they were intended to do.) Subsequently conducted surveys, to learn whether such a revision in policy would impact donors' decisions to contribute to sperm banks, revealed a desire among donors to remain anonymous. The United States is distinctive in that egg and sperm donation occurs both anonymously and nonanonymously. Anonymity is still the norm, despite legislation motivated by ethical concerns to make the process one in which identities are revealed. For a discussion about the secrecy surrounding donor insemination and the problems that emerge from this practice, see Paul Lauritzen, *Pursuing Parenthood: Ethical Issues in Assisted Reproduction* (Bloomington: Indiana University Press, 1993), 79–89. For information on the demographic backgrounds of sperm donors and their desire to remain anonymous, see U. Van den Broeck, "A Systematic Review of Sperm Donors: Demographic Characteristics, Attitudes, Motives, and Experiences of the Process of Sperm Donation," http://humupd.oxfordjournals.org/content/19/1/37.full.

26. Healy, *Last Best Gifts*, 116.

27. Ibid., 116.

28. Courtney Bender, *Heaven's Kitchen: Living Religion at God's Love We Deliver* (Chicago: University of Chicago Press, 2003), also discussed by Healy, *Last Best Gifts*, 116–17.

29. Healy, *Last Best Gifts*, 15; italics in original. See also Marcel Mauss, *The Gift: The Form and Reason for Exchange in Archaic Societies* (New York: Norton, 2000); and Bronislaw Malinowski, *Crime and Custom in Savage Society* (London: Routledge, 1926).

30. Bruno S. Frey, Felix Oberholzer-Gee, and Reiner Eichenberger, "The Old Lady Visits Your Backyard: A Tale of Morals and Markets," *Journal of Political Economy* 104, no. 6 (December 1996): 1297–1313; and Bruno S. Frey and Felix Oberholzer-Gee, "The Cost of Price Incentives: An Empirical Analysis of Motivation Crowding-Out," *American Economic Review* 87, no. 4 (September 1997): 746–55.

31. Richard M. Titmuss, *The Gift Relationship: From Human Blood to Social Policy* (New York: Vintage, 1971), 177, 223–24.

32. Ali R. Ahmadi et al., "Shifting Paradigms in Eligibility Criteria for Live Kidney Donation: A Systematic Review," *Kidney International* 87, no. 1 (2015): 31–45.

1

The Case for Legalizing the Sale of Organs

THE MARKET AS A SOLUTION, IF NOT A VIRTUE

Since 1984, when the National Organ Transplantation Act (NOTA) laid the groundwork for a national procurement and transplantation network to match organ donors with recipients, it has been illegal in the United States for "any person to knowingly acquire, receive, or otherwise transfer any human organ for valuable consideration for use in human transplantation if the transfer affects interstate commerce."[1] It is significant that from the moment it became legal to donate an organ, the deed was defined as a gift. That a donor cannot be paid is, historically, a big reason that organ transplantation came to acquire widespread public acceptance. It is by virtue of this proscription that eleven years after NOTA passed, Pope John Paul II urged Catholics to consider organ donation as part of "the culture of life."[2] Following his endorsement, the Anglican Church and leaders of denominations of other major traditions followed suit, all citing similar rationales based on a religious obligation to help the neighbor.[3] Just a few years after its enactment, NOTA signaled the realization of overdue and hopeful legislation for those chronically on dialysis, not only by raising the possibility of a new medical alternative for those suffering from end-stage renal disease (ESRD) but also in affirming the sacrosanct adage of medicine that one ought not to profit from another's suffering.

There are other reasons why legislation that prohibited the introduction of money into the exchange arose at the same time as when society first came to terms with organ donation as accepted medical practice. First, medical ethicists and healthcare practitioners were worried about safety. Remembering the history of blood donation and the reason for the decision to allow no longer the sale of blood in the United States, they were worried that a market for profit on organs would induce potential donors to lie when reporting on their social histories and fail to mention their existing medical conditions. Second, allowing donors to be paid raised questions about free and informed consent, particularly in the case of impoverished or desperate individuals volunteering to give their body parts to recipients of means. If organs were for sale, then how could procurement organizations overseeing the exchange be sure that donors could be guaranteed to give them to needy recipients in a manner free of coercion?[4] Third, concerns about commodification of the human body surfaced in connection with a whole class of goods thought to be "sacred" in the era of science and technology: What were the consequences, many wondered, of making for sale that over which only God could claim ownership?

These concerns made the acceptance of organ donation in the late 1980s and 1990s contingent upon buy-in on the part of religious leaders, who remained theologically uncomfortable about reducing the exchange of organs to a contractual transaction. Advocates for transplantation ultimately overcame a recalcitrant and maybe even squeamish public by casting organ donation as a noble, virtuous path that opened a special I-Thou relationship between donor and recipient. Once accepting the blessing of religious leaders, the transplantation industry became, in a sense, a victim of its own success.[5] It was believed that adding a financial incentive would undermine the basis on which organ donation first came to legitimacy and effectively treat much of the public like fools whose sentiments could be easily manipulated. In this historical light, it is not surprising that over the last forty years a number of significant policy statements have emerged to shape the consensus both abroad and here at home to uphold the intuition that organ donation should be seen strictly as a gift and not a part of commerce. Prominent nongovernmental organizations and state-funded institutions, including the Transplantation Society, the World Health Organization, the US Task Force on Organ Transplantation, the National Kidney Foundation, the United Network for Organ Sharing (UNOS), and the US Congress, have all supported the proscription against selling organs.[6]

The most thoughtful proponents of creating a market for organ trade acknowledge the concerns their critics raise but note that things have changed since 1984 in terms of both the urgency of the matter at hand and our ability to address anew the ethical and practical misgivings underlying them. Through the means of careful regulation, which proponents claim has never been fully attempted, most concerns about safety, exploitation, and commodification can now be answered.

One of the biggest problems with the way the issue has been historically framed, according to proponents, is that in a market the procurement and allocation processes are understood to be linked. Allowing for the sale of organs need not invite scenarios in which organ donors receive lump-sum payments directly from their recipients. A properly regulated market could create a reserve bank of funds, presumably from the same state or national sources for which dialysis expenses are presently reimbursed, and this, in turn, could be earmarked for compensating a donor for his or her generous sacrifice. It is important to keep in mind the proponents' stated motivations for their call to reform: the needs of desperate recipients must be addressed, and donors should be adequately compensated for their sacrifice. The nature of the objections raised are substantive but, proponents point out, they are more problematic in the context of the black or underground market than in a properly regulated one. Proponents seek to introduce a regulated market as the *alternative* to the black one. They are also aware that the practice of selling organs ignores a presumptively inviolable proscription against commodifying something rightly reserved for the altruistic sphere. Their response to this reservation is that the one opposed to the creation of a market had better have good reason other than just popular mythology behind the objection. With so much at stake, stereotypes will not suffice to solve an organ shortage problem growing out of control.

Transplant surgeons, free market economists, and some medical ethicists want to improve the lives and contributions to society of those currently on dialysis who could receive a new kidney, but they hold that in order to do so we must appreciate that human beings are motivated by capitalist incentives. They argue that without sufficient *and* the right sort of compensation we will be hard-pressed to convince people to make such a considerable sacrifice for someone. This approach assumes markets are self-correcting by nature, making them optimally efficient. Scarcity, not preciousness, is what principally brings about demand. As such, creating a market for a good that is in *scarce* supply, and thereby viewing that scarce good as a commodity that is subject to fluctuating value like any other item for sale, is the most efficient way of affecting that good when it is in short supply, even if it is a good to which we happen to attach intangible value.

Proponents of creating a market for transplantation of bodily organs also care about treating comparable issues equitably. They urge us to consider comparisons between organ donors, on the one hand, and donors of egg and sperm (who can legally be paid), on the other, as well as to consider surrogacy,

military service, and other circumstances where society handsomely acknowledges, through monetary compensation, the sacrificer who incurs costs in
pursuit of a larger altruistic objective. They maintain that the practice of assigning sacred status is fraught with the danger of imposing one's own value
system. Why is one good off-limits to assigning a monetary equivalence, but
not another? Proponents of creating a market for organ trade see themselves
as nonpolitical within a market that is designed precisely to avoid arbitrary
evaluations. It is concerned only with efficiently replenishing a scarce but
vital good.

Those in favor of creating a market for organ trade distinguish between
a principle that specifies the limits within which good policy can be created
and good policy itself, the only constraint of which is to solve the current
problem in the best possible way. Since NOTA was passed, the waiting time
for a kidney has grown. To those expressing concern that if kidneys were for
sale, the rich, white, or privileged recipient might take advantage of the poor
or people of color, proponents note that the ones who wait the longest are
disproportionately African Americans and individuals otherwise lacking in
resources. Best intentions often lead to the worst outcomes.

Proscription justified by ethical principle alone amounts to aloof moralism, not because legitimate ethical misgivings cannot be identified but because they should not trump what ought to be seen as the most important
ethical consideration at stake: the well-being of the donor and the recipient.[7]
"Those who are opposed to a regulated system of sales," writes Dr. Arthur
Matas, a surgeon at the University of Minnesota, "imply that they are taking
the moral high ground by protecting the potential paid donor (from exploitation? from the harm of surgery?) or by protecting society (from the loss of
human dignity?). The end result, however, is that they are sentencing many
of our transplant candidates to death."[8]

As Robert Kuttner notes, it is the purpose of all markets to discover, naturally, what works with the greatest efficiency. Without demonstrating that a
contractual arrangement would lead to some other pragmatic disbenefit, such
as a widespread erosion of trust in society, it ought to become the default
solution to a problem if idealistic proposals have fallen short. Market theory
conceives of economic relationships as instrumental to making a good available. "All transactions are at an arm's length," Kuttner explains, "and there is
no room for sentimentality."[9] To be opposed to using a market solution to
correct the gap between supply and demand, one must make an independent
pragmatic argument that a particular economic relationship ought to be *more*

than instrumental and that replenishing a specific scarce good is somehow tied to a perception of that good that should not be reduced to its tangible component. Granted, the perception of the relationship between organ donor and recipient historically has been construed as spiritual in nature, which bonds the two parties together in a sacred common cause. Because of unprecedented exigency, however, the time has come to revisit this assumption.

If kidney donors would be better off maximizing their options, including having additional means of income if they are impoverished, and if recipients would be better off having to wait less time than they currently do to receive a new kidney, then we must ask: What is the real pay-off in insisting that donation not be rewarded with money? Is it just to maintain the "purity" of the gift? In order to be truly virtuous, virtue must be in service of a solution. When taken together, the various strands of argumentation in favor of a market approach buttress one essential claim: in an era when a regulated and safely administered market for organ exchange could theoretically be developed, it is antiquated moralism rather than legitimate problem-solving to disallow the introduction of money into the exchange.

COSTS AND EQUITY

Proponents and opponents of creating a market for legalizing the sale of organs disagree about which incentives are the most powerful for motivating human behavior. But they concur that giving one's kidney is a wonderful and selfless gesture made all the more remarkable because it comes with certain risks and possibly significant costs to the donor. Besides the pain and inconvenience created in one's life from the surgery itself (two to six weeks of discomfort from bloating, not carrying anything greater than ten pounds in that time, and the financial burdens associated with the disruption in his or her work schedule), there are significant long-term implications of being a living donor. With a mortality rate of 3 per 10,000 and a complication rate of 1–2 percent (and hospital readmission less than 1 percent), a nephrectomy is among the safest "not necessary" surgery one can undergo. Even when everything does go as planned, however, the donor is choosing to do something not in his or her own best medical interests for the sake of another person.

As with all surgeries requiring the suppression of the central nervous system, nephrectomies entail life-threatening risks and complications, including allergic reaction to general anesthesia, pneumonia, the formation of blood clots in the lungs, infections around the points of incision and organ(s) targeted for removal, and internal bleeding. Following a nephrectomy, one goes from having 100 percent of one's kidney function to only half that, and over time increasing to only about 65–70 percent function, as the remaining kidney picks up some of the freight formerly carried by the absent one. Because organ donors are among the healthiest individuals among us, their risk of acquiring end-stage renal disease following a nephrectomy is no greater than the general population, but a donor may incur an increased risk of high blood pressure, particularly if he or she has a family history of hypertension or is even mildly obese—two factors that, in turn, increase risk for heart attack and stroke.[10]

Some evidence shows a higher risk for depression among donors. Additionally, a donor must commit to maintaining a healthy lifestyle for the remainder of his or her life, to monitoring the consumption of alcohol and prescription drugs, to avoiding anti-inflammatory medications like ibuprofen (which are processed in the kidney), to being vigilant about participating in contact sports and watching sugar intake. It is possible that donating one's kidney heightens one's risk for developing type 2 diabetes (which is already the leading cause of kidney failure) as well as lower-limb amputations (other than those caused by injury) and new cases of blindness among adults.[11] Nephrectomies among living donors are still too new to be able to draw reliable conclusions about a correlation between them and the development of type 2 diabetes years later, but living donor coordinators privately acknowledge this as one of their primary concerns. It is certainly something that living donor advocates mention to donors when procuring their consent prior to surgery. This is all to suggest that we are nowhere near a point in time in which we can expect an individual to have the luxury of being able to give his or her kidney to a needy recipient and then nonchalantly go back to life undisturbed. For the recipient *and* the donor, things will have changed forever.

Those who advocate for monetarily compensating donors infer from the costs that it would be exploitation not to acknowledge tangibly the donors' significant sacrifice. Their reasoning is similar to veteran advocates, who want us never to forget individuals who put themselves in harm's way so that the rest of are safe. We pay pensions, provide higher education, supply health care, and offer other benefits to those who have served in the military as a way both of acknowledging their sacrifice and recruiting future volunteers. By the same token, society allows a surrogate mother to get paid for lending her uterus to another couple for over nine months, the last days of which carry known medical risks and are in any case uncomfortable for the surrogate. We allow sperm and egg donors to be compensated for their contributions to future parents who desperately want to have children. Beyond these examples, there is ample precedent in the current American system of medicine, even in the era of the Affordable Care Act, for practitioners, healthcare providers, and insurers to profit from the services they render, including instances in which we pay for "enhanced" services not covered through the normal means of reimbursement. Some physicians command a retainer to be on call in a private setting for select, elite patients, while many plastic surgeons get paid directly from their patients for performing cosmetic surgeries.[12] Why, among all of these examples, is paying a living organ donor legally proscribed? Isn't such discrimination tantamount to imposing a double standard by elevating the organ donor to some sort of sainthood while others are allowed to benefit for the goods and services they render? The principle of equity, it seems, would dictate that we ought to be allowed to pay the organ donor too.

In response to this argument, some say that it would be predatory to pay organ donors whose desperation for cash might cloud their ability to think through their consent and weigh the costs involved in their decision. Proponents are receptive to this point, but the objection remains: Why single out the organ donor? Writing in an opinion piece for the *New York Times* days before he was to give his kidney to someone he'd never met, Alexander Berger reflects:

> Last week, the Ninth Circuit Court of Appeals issued a ruling legalizing compensation for bone marrow donors; we already allow paid plasma, sperm and egg donation, as well as payment for surrogate mothers. Contrary to early fears that paid surrogacy would exploit young, poor minority women, most surrogate mothers are married, middle class and white; the evidence suggests that, far from trying to "cash in," they take pride in performing a service that brings others great happiness. And we regularly pay people to take socially beneficial but physically dangerous jobs—soldiers, police officers and firefighters all earn a living while risking their lives—without worrying that they are taken advantage of.[13]

Not only is there an exclusion that applies to donors, who unlike the others just mentioned are barred from being compensated, there is also an equity issue internal to the living donation process itself. As Amy Friedman notes, besides the recipients themselves, who obviously benefit,

> their family members [enjoy] extra income if the recipient returns to work. Doctors will be paid for each transplantation. And other hospital staff, such as administrators and transplant coordinators, whose jobs depend on the volume of transplantations, will validate their effectiveness by satisfying job requirements. Transplant programmes and their home institutions gain higher case volumes, which improves their reputation and gives them a competitive advantage. Taxpayers might also benefit financially because the support of a kidney transplant recipient is less costly than haemodialysis or peritoneal dialysis. Furthermore, many recipients will restart work and pay taxes. In contrast, living donors are prohibited by law from receiving "valuable consideration" in exchange for their gift.[14]

Aside from immediate donor care, which is typically covered by a recipient's insurance, donors are not allowed to receive any money for their gift and must bear travel costs, suffer the brunt of lost wages, and manage the cost of possible long-term complications that cannot directly be linked to the nephrectomy but may well have something to do with it. To preserve the sanctity of their heroism, donors, ironically, become the only ones in the donation process for whom the deed remains a burden. Raising the example of human subjects who volunteer for medical trials and experiments, Friedman notes that were it not for our ability to compensate these individuals, we would likely never be able to recruit them.[15] What would happen to new, lifesaving technologies on which medical practitioners and society rely if we could not pay such volunteers?

Adding to this argument for equity, Mark Cherry maintains that there is a difference in treatment between the many occasions on which renderers of a costly good are permitted to avail themselves of the principle of autonomy and profit from an opportunity that could greatly improve their living situation, and the one instance when this natural right is denied. Cherry argues that it is an arbitrary imposition to deny an individual authority over his or her own body or to limit that individual's ability to engage in his or her own prudential reasoning process whereby he or she will remain free to come to an assessment of what constitutes the final say on overall benefits and harms.[16]

This kind of proscription is based on a well-entrenched tradition in medical ethics to provide the greatest protection to the most helpless or financially needy individuals who might shortsightedly be induced to part with one of their kidneys. But such paternalism, even when well-intended, selectively punishes the one who is about to engage in the most impactful and noble display of self-sacrifice. This makes the presumed norm not only unequal but also doubly unfair. Cherry agrees with his critics, that life doesn't begin on a level playing field for all, that all don't labor under the same handicaps in terms of trying to secure basic conditions for their flourishing, and that some will always be more vulnerable than others.

The empirical reality that our set of inherited hardships differ from one another, however, should collectively serve to open up, not limit, opportunities to the ones most struggling (for example, to the poor who strive to emerge from poverty). Cherry is aware of Michael Walzer's misgiving, that a market blind to the concrete hardships of diverse groups lacks the inherent ability to put every prospective participant on equal footing and therefore fails to have the ability "to approximate an exchange between equals."[17]

Supporting Walzer's view, Joel Feinberg emphasizes the inherently exploitative nature of any transaction in which one party benefits to a significantly greater degree than the other, even if both marginally benefit in the end.[18] Precisely this concern expressed by Walzer and Feinberg came to pass in India, where selling one's kidney was legal until 1994. In a study conducted in Chennai, India, an area known to be replete with debtors, researchers found that those who sold their kidneys to repay what they owed lenders were given neither enough to get out of their current debts nor enough to stay clear of a debt-free existence in the long run.[19] In a desperate moment, when one is not necessarily thinking clearly, one is not likely to split hairs about whether or not his interests are being fully or fairly considered prior to the transaction. Getting the deal done in a timely fashion is more important.

Cherry's reply calls attention to the difference between a regulated and an unregulated market. The state could, if it wanted, adjust the price of a kidney to redress the concern expressed by Walzer and Feinberg, that both parties' interests be equitably addressed. That it didn't happen in India during the time in which selling organs was legal is no argument that it couldn't ever happen.[20] To the heart of the objection, Cherry points out the shortsightedness of a paternalism that trades on a preemptive protection. Such an approach, he argues, offers safeguards against possible but not always evident exploitation by guaranteeing that the relative well-being of the one protected gets *neither* worse nor better:

While such policies may prima facie appear less exploitative, they have counterintuitive consequences. First, they further restrict options for the poor; second, unlike those better off, the impoverished are prevented from fully utilizing the market for their own advantage. While a poor individual may decide that selling a kidney is more attractive than other options, offers to purchase an organ do not make him worse off if he refuses to sell. Analogously, on the labor market, those who must settle for any unpleasant or more risky occupation, such as ditch digging, oil-platform construction, assembly-line worker, and so on, must make the same type of choice; this does not necessarily mean that they are being coerced.[21]

Why is donating an organ to better one's lot in life thought to be more institutionally coercive than taking a labor-intensive job replete with occupational hazards for the same reason? Much is built into the notion that organ donation is relevantly like the other sorts of examples he mentions, and Cherry is convincing to the degree that he persuades that the analogy is apt. We do not question the permissibility of taking risks for profit in order to make a living in one sort of case, so we shouldn't in the other. We will later examine whether these examples are in fact analogous, but it bears noting that Cherry and others seem to reject out of hand a qualifier that *any* particular good is more "especially precious" such that it warrants restrictive oversight on the part of some larger body that knows what is best for the individual whose decision it actually is to take part in a proposed exchange.

Cherry makes a distinction between "coercion," which illegitimately forces individuals into a disadvantage, and "peaceable manipulation," in which opportunities present themselves when one is already at a disadvantage at the time one comes to the situation.[22] The latter, according to Cherry, neither violates an individual's autonomy of free choice nor illegitimately places that individual in any *additional* harm. According to this analysis, creating a market for the sale of organs would be a win-win for both recipient and donor, assuming that the donor is fully informed about risks and potential costs and has at all times the full power to refuse any offer placed before him or her. As Robert Veatch and Lainie Ross note,

Assuming that the vendor is an adult who is mentally competent and has been informed adequately about the risks and benefits of selling a kidney, and assuming that this person, after careful consideration, comes to the conclusion that it is better to sell the kidney and do something with the money, why should our society prohibit such sales? It cannot be that such persons have always calculated their interests incorrectly. Some people really would be better off with the money than with the second kidney (or they may be able to act more morally—taking care of loved ones in desperate need). If we are going to make such sales illegal, we need an argument that overrules the enlightened self-interest of such sellers.[23]

Assuming responsible oversight in any transaction between donor (or vendor) and recipient—and Cherry, Veatch, and Ross are happy to stipulate that such an assumption is crucial—then creating a market for organ trade should be regarded as no more than giving both recipient and donor an option that they previously didn't have. Who better than these two parties (and not a third party) to know what is in their own best interests?

The critic might grant the legitimacy of the comparisons Cherry and others draw between vitally rendered goods that entail high costs but still reject the proposal to legalize the sale of organs. Perhaps the other examples the proponent lists (egg and sperm donation, surrogacy, military service, other service-oriented pursuits that involve occupational hazards) are *also* the type of things in which we should offer protections in the context of a market. Just because society is laissez-faire with regard to an activity of commerce doesn't mean it *should* be so hands off. Let's consider one of the most interesting examples mentioned here: surrogacy.

It is currently legal for a couple from the West to pay between six and seven thousand dollars to procure the services of a woman from India to carry its baby to term, which is about a third to a fourth of the legal going rate in the United States. This is interesting for purposes of our current discussion because it is well known how onerous pregnancy can be and, similar to living donation, one's planned sacrifice might jeopardize a healthy life currently under way. The poor, in particular, are vulnerable to both sorts of commodification. As Margaret Jane Radin observes, paid surrogacy places the socioeconomically disadvantaged in a "double bind": the mere possibility of getting paid to carry another couple's baby to term puts the surrogate between a rock and a hard place, where, in a worst-case scenario, "rich women, even those who are not infertile, might employ poor women to bear children for them," while the prospective surrogate may not have the luxury to refuse the offer, given that she has others who depend on her and even if doing so appears degrading.[24] The case of paid surrogacy is arguably *more* complicated and *more* morally problematic than paying a living donor.

Gender is also a factor in the case of paid surrogacy since women, in particular their reproductive capacities and their genes, become "fungible in carrying on the male genetic line."[25] Poor women might be drawn to the opportunity because it allows them to fulfill a gender role to which they imagine they are natively suited, but when doing so for hire, their intended role as nurturer and caretaker can become inverted and assume an oppressive character.[26] Poor or not, there is an emotional bond that naturally forms between mother and baby. Whether surrogacy leads to long-term psychological damage that severs this bond is just beginning to be understood adequately as surrogacy enters the sphere of commerce in greater incidence.

None of this, furthermore, acknowledges that a new life hangs in the balance, the caring for which doesn't necessarily but possibly could by virtue of the contractual arrangement become confusing for all the parties involved. What if something goes wrong with the pregnancy and all of the adults involved abdicate responsibility for the child?[27] In cases where good people appeal to the public to help them conceive, there are no doubt wonderful benefits to the service a surrogate renders. But, as with organ donation, the overall process has high stakes and is a rather big deal for the one who decides to carry the fetus to term.

Certainly, bringing somebody else's baby to term *is* analogous to donating one's organ and may be an even more costly endeavor for the sacrificing party and give more fuel to the claim that making a sale legal in one case and not in the other is not equitable treatment. The asymmetry begs further questions. What is the relative value society places on the pursuit of parenthood versus the transitioning of 100,000 citizens off of dialysis?[28] Under what conditions can a human body's use be deemed able to be commodified, and on whose authority is such a judgment made? Our society has legislatively evolved to harbor few reservations about resorting to capitalistic incentives in order to perpetuate a culture of life in the realm of procreation. Maybe if we became more aware of the crisis and the growing gap between available organs and needy recipients we wouldn't be so resistant to pragmatic solutions.

Opponents of relaxing the prohibition against organ sales may respond emotionally to this appeal to equity but interpret the observation not as a justification for the creation of a market for organ trade but rather about the arbitrary and morally problematic way in which we decide it is okay to resort to commodification in many instances. Why not correct for the disparity by disallowing commodification across the board? We here arrive at the fundamental question about what kind of society we are and whether capitalism is the best system for incentivizing the perpetuation of tangible outcomes with intangible relevance. It seems at least plausible to suggest that, right or wrong, it is discriminatory against the organ donor to (1) allow others in society relevantly circumstanced to profit from their sacrifices on behalf of a greater good and (2) allow everyone *besides* the donor to benefit from the organ donation process, including OPOs, transplant surgeons, healthcare-providing institutions with transplantation facilities, and the recipients themselves. One breach in the dike and the floodgates have opened. The system currently in place, sanctioned from its inception in 1984 that transplantations can occur only in conditions of unpaid consent, is inherently unstable so long as it stands alongside markets for qualitatively similar goods that are allowed to flourish unchecked.

THE "TYRANNY OF THE GIFT"

The exploration of the case for legalization has so far centered on the interests of the donor. The proponent makes a strong point that the donor seems discriminated against, given the social context of other individuals poised to serve society in similar ways. According to proponents, however, the donor's perspective is not the only one to consider when making a case for legalization. They also direct our attention to what life looks like from the vantage point of those who desperately need to find someone else to step up so that they are not consigned to life on dialysis unto death.

Customarily, one's family provides this volunteer. It stands to reason that one's family would be especially motivated to do so: a family member not only presumably loves the recipient but is also the most biologically suited, in terms of blood type and antibodies, to donate. Unfortunately, one's family members cannot always be depended on to be a biological match, and in some cases not even depended on to be motivated from kinship to give away a kidney even if they are a match. Besides biological incompatibility, a number of other things can get in the way of one's plan to depend on one's family member(s). Often such complications don't manifest themselves until time is running out and prospective donors are unexpectedly placed in the position of having to make a rushed decision. To mention but one example, I came across a case of a young woman in need of a kidney whose sibling was a perfect match, but her mother insisted that both of her children not be under anesthesia at the same time. (The family took to Facebook to attempt to recruit a donor from the local public.) There are often long-standing rifts of a personal nature between family members, which the pressure of an individual with a failing kidney only exacerbates. Sometimes it is the potential recipient who refuses to place himself or herself in lifelong debt to the family member who would otherwise serve as the only suitable match.

Genetically speaking, siblings comprise the most ideal donors, but not all individuals in need of kidneys have siblings. In lieu of willing-and-able siblings, the situation becomes trickier for a donor relying on his or her family. One reason for this is that it is not always medically appropriate for someone from a younger generation to donate to someone who is older, even if that person is a blood relative.[29] Thus, while in some cultures there is an expectation that a son or daughter, or even a grandson or granddaughter, will without any discussion volunteer to save the life of an elder family member, living donor coordinators have to make sure that the decision is truly voluntarily made in order to abide the guideline of informed consent. For good reason such candidates are often ruled out. Overall, finding a donor from among one's blood relatives is for a number of reasons not always simple.

In cases where donors cannot be recruited from one's biological family (or one's spouse or partner), the recipient is left scrambling to find a willing benefactor from among his or her larger circle of friends and acquaintances. This too contains its own drawbacks. What happens to a friendship when one makes this kind of ask? If it is not a close friendship, where does one find the wherewithal to muster the rapport even to raise the issue? Someone in need of a kidney might find herself having to search for a willing donor and not know where to begin. Bereft of the help of a market that might have incentivized a biologically suitable stranger to step up, recipients face the prospect of jeopardizing relationships that are important to them. In these cases actual capital is preserved at the expense of social capital, thereby adding the proverbial insult (feeling isolated) to injury (one's failing kidneys).

In 2005 Dr. Sally Satel, a psychiatrist in her late forties, found herself in this position. In lieu of being able to identify someone from her family, she became desperate to find a different living donor who was willing to help her. Describing her new life facing imminent dialysis in which for much of the week she would have to be "tethered to a machine" for four "debilitating" hours at a time, Satel chronicled her experience, where stranger after stranger led her down the garden path, promising to be her donor savior but then backing out at the eleventh hour.[30] After disappointment after crushing disappointment, Satel began to resent being so completely at the mercy of someone who could, without providing a reason, change his or her mind. In each instance a potential donor would appear, seemingly out of nowhere, and then disappear just as suddenly. To hear Satel describe it, the experience of waiting for a kidney sounds horrendous. Even in the few superficial conversations she had with potential donors she felt she had to monitor everything she said lest she accidentally utter something to offend or give that person pause.

There were other unpleasantries as well: weighing the prospect of being indebted to a stranger and wanting to reciprocate for something that is impossible to reciprocate; existing as the helpless party in a two-person dynamic; and coming to realize, just days following pretesting, that the promise she received was no longer valid and the one promising would never be heard from again. Reflecting on her experience prior to the time when a kidney came through for her from the least likely of sources, Satel invokes a term first introduced in 1992 by medical sociologists Renée C. Fox and Judith P. Swazey: the "tyranny of the gift." As Fox and Swazey explain, in the grip of such tyranny the "giver, the receiver, and their families may find themselves locked in a creditor-debtor vise that binds them to one another in a mutually fettering way."[31] This assessment is striking in its irony, since the creditor-debtor dynamic is the very thing that opponents to legalizing the sale of organs aim to avoid by abolishing the contractual feature of a negotiation at the outset of the discussion. The most heartbreaking of the successive broken promises with which Satel had to contend came at the hand of a Canadian man who, she remembers, was particularly convincing when he first expressed his desire to be her donor. Quickly after meeting him, however, she could sense she was walking on eggshells:

> Although the Canadian seemed kind and steady, he had enormous power over me. I deliberately kept our calls brief to minimize my chances of saying something that might antagonize him. I wondered why he chose me, but I dared not ask, lest his decision was based on a misconception of who I was. Would I then be morally bound to set him straight so that he wasn't giving a body part under false pretenses? What if he loathed conservatives? After all, he was involved in politics, and I was associated with a right-of-center think tank.[32]

Satel's lived experience as an awaiting recipient, combined with her awareness of the exponentially growing shortage (far worse now than when she wrote this editorial), ultimately led her to conclude, despite her eventual fortunate ending, that a desperate predicament that depends on altruism for its solution falls "painfully short of its goal." Far from exacerbating an unjust power dynamic, contractual arrangements based on financial incentives represent the best means of putting both parties on an equal level.

Satel introduces to this discussion a disturbing idea that she could have absorbed only through experience: perhaps it is *altruism* that becomes coercive when institutionalized, rather than the opposite. From the perspective of the one on dialysis, the miracle of being graced by another's saving gesture is but a shallow ideal if it puts the recipient in the position of playing the beggar. Apparently, "near-transplant experiences" are not uncommon. And although transplantations tend to bring the donor and recipient closer together, from time to time the experience has been known to destroy relationships, even between family members.[33] Without a financial contract in place, according to Satel, both parties will tend to harbor tacit expectations of the other. Recipients must cope with a state of being eternally beholden to donors, while donors, who have just given away something precious without being compensated, can only pray that the recipient will be a responsible steward of the gift bestowed.

These expectations do not always match up with reality. A gift, once given, is no longer the possession of the giver, and all too frequently, as living transplant coordinators can painfully attest, a recipient will disrespect the second chance on life he or she has been given by failing to take the prescribed regimen of immunosuppressant drugs or by drinking alcohol more than he or she should, or by other sorts of negligence. This is, of course, tragic when it occurs. But if what has been received is truly a *gift*, there is probably nothing that can be done in advance to guarantee that such an outcome won't come to pass.

Satel raises the notion that such perils arise specifically in the context of our current system in which the sale of organs is disallowed. By contrast, contractual arrangements of a financial nature with clearly stated impersonal guidelines that are introduced at the time of the exchange replace the potential for either the giving or the receiving party to be beleaguered psychologically by the host of expectations that may arise. Along the lines of this thinking, one has grounds to conclude that a financial arrangement is both cleaner and freer of messy human entanglements captured by scenarios involving the transfer of substantial gifts. Contracts that exactly specify which rewards are earned through sacrifice leave to no one's imagination what is expected to transpire. Such exactitude does cap the potential boundless nature of one's grace. However, to the extent that a system of exchange that relies on market incentives is pessimistic about the appearance of our better angels, it is a realistic approach to solving big problems where precious goods lay in demand. If nothing else, contractual arrangements protect against the realization of the worst-case scenario in which one gives the impression he or she will come to the rescue of another and then fails to live up to this promise.

FINANCIAL INCENTIVES, LIBERTARIANISM, AND THE BLACK MARKET

The two sorts of arguments made so far on behalf of legalizing the sale of organs have been essentially of a negative character. First is that the costs entailed in nephrectomies are too great to pin our hopes reliably on uncompensated volunteers, an argument given fuel by the reality that in comparable circumstances involving other precious goods, the one sacrificing *is* compensated. Second is the psychologically oppressive nature of identifying a precious good as a gift, since such a designation confers on the exchange an inappropriate power dynamic that saddles both giver and recipient with undue pressure to play an assigned role. It is now time to make the positive case on behalf of the proponent for legalization.

Like Amy Friedman, most transplant surgeons who publicly make the case for the creation of a legal market for organ trade tend to focus on the shortsighted wisdom of "waiting with dignity for the organ that never comes." Their philosophical allies, free-market economists, proceed by insisting that there is no real distinction between kinds of goods in demand. Bodily organs are in essence no different than "burgers or candy"—that is, they are tradable items eligible for purchase that ought to require only a willing and freely consenting seller and an equally willing buyer. So claims the medical ethicist and libertarian James Stacey Taylor.[34] In fact, the *more* in demand a particular good is, the more the construing of it as a commodity with a natural selling price like any other commodity stands to alleviate the gap between supply and demand. In situations marked by disparity, which always make the shortages of precious goods more conspicuous, poverty, not markets, remains the underlying problem.[35]

This assessment goes to a fundamental commitment about what many libertarians think underlies human motivation and human freedom: the voluntary nature of autonomous decision-making to evaluate for oneself what represents the best solution to one's own idiosyncratic set of problems. A default policy of universal commodification sees the individual in the first instance as a "commodity trader," or a decider of one's own interests and pursuits in which one is allowed to advocate on behalf of oneself with minimal restrictions. A society of commodity traders is one in which everyone is presumably equally unrestricted and therefore everyone collectively benefits to the greatest degree. That we are hardwired to be self-interested is not a decision up to us; the libertarian views it as a presumed fact of human existence. Markets merely represent the most efficient economic appropriation of this fact. Margaret Jane Radin elaborates on the political and economic implications of such a worldview:

> All social and political interactions are conceived of as exchanges for monetizable gains. Politics reduces to "rent seeking" by logrolling selfish individuals or groups, in which those individuals or groups vie to capture social wealth for themselves. The social ideal reduces to efficiency. Efficiency is pursued through the market methodology of cost-benefit analysis. Cost-benefit analysis evaluates human actions and social outcomes in terms of actual or hypothetical gains from trade, measured in money. In seeking efficiency through market methodology, universal commodification posits the laissez-faire market as the rule.[36]

The laissez-faire approach, clarifies Radin, is presumed to be efficient because of its system of voluntary transfers, which, given universal commodification, both maximizes gains from trade and optimally upholds expressions of freedom. Whether I want a hamburger at the local diner or I am desperately in need of a kidney from an anonymous donor, no one is more acutely aware of my current or long-term needs than I am. My dignity is bound up in nothing as much as my deliberate and self-determined pursuit to satisfy these needs. To the extent that I am presented with needless obstacles that hinder my realizing the ends I determine for myself, I am stripped of that which makes me most myself. Associations into which we interdependently enter with others may from time to time reflect our best means of fulfilling our needs, but we are essentially on our own when presented with the prospect of vital goods in need of replenishment: nobody knows better than we do what we ought to try to acquire. Enforceable guidelines can be essential to our pursuit of goods, or of our good generally, but only to the extent that they facilitate rather than restrict this endeavor.

In this way of thinking it becomes arrogance of the first degree for a third party to intervene and decide what is in the best interest of two adults poised to enter into a transaction. Taylor, in his writings, interviews, and YouTube videos, is fond of pointing out the extent to which common sense is on his side. In one of his go-to anecdotes, he recalls the story of Peter Randall, who in 2003 offered his kidney for sale on eBay: "He wasn't doing this as a publicity stunt or because he was greedy and wanted a new Ferrari. He was doing it because he thought it was the only way in which he could raise enough money to pay for the therapy of his daughter, Alice, who at the time was six years old and suffering from cerebral palsy."[37] Randall received at least three serious offers from people living in the United States alone, despite the fact that (as they presumably knew) it is currently illegal in this country to engage in this sort of transaction. That Randall immediately found willingly interested parties in the arena of the black market testifies all the more to the potential for a legitimate market for organ trade to flourish. To deny individuals the opportunity to decide what is in their best interests is to add momentum to an underground locus for organ trade that, all agree, *is* dangerous and *does* imperil the already vulnerable. The argument is similar to those made by pro-rights activists, who note that desperately poor women who need to end their pregnancies will find one way or another to do so. By disallowing a legitimate market within which to conduct a needed transaction, the black market becomes the only remaining viable option for determined seekers of a good or service.

Proponents of legalizing the sale of organs are the first to agree that the black market—in which, de facto, the sale of organs does take place—is no solution at all. The black market has no guarantee of clean surgical equipment and sterile operating conditions; no post-op follow-up appointments with physicians to monitor the progress of both donors and recipients; no individual whose role in the process is to serve as an independent advocate for the donor to make sure he or she is not being exploited; no medications, such as immunosuppressant drugs that allow the recipient not to reject the transplanted organ; and no expectation on the part of either party that what is paid or received reflects that which would reasonably be considered a fair value. In terms of this last feature, there are often so many middlemen who stand to profit in brokering an illegal kidney sale, for example, that the donor and recipient are often both exploited.[38] The safety and financial protection of both concerned parties are not only neglected in the black market; they are blatantly subverted. This is because of the inherent conflict of interest on the part of brokers who, without being compelled to act differently by any regulating body or governmental agency, have no incentive to bear the extra costs associated with providing protections. Finally, if the organ trade is occurring underground, we lack the reliable means to monitor adverse outcomes that donors or recipients may experience.[39] It is estimated that the black market for the trade of organs imperils several hundred thousand people around the world. People who sell their kidneys endure the risk of undergoing surgery with untrained practitioners, suffer infections, and bear the consequence of criminal prosecution if they are discovered to have broken the law.[40] Disturbingly, if not surprisingly, there is no evidence that any of these realities serve as disincentives to people who are desperate to find replacements for their failing kidneys. Desperation has its own logic.

A black market, however, is not a regulated market, and to libertarians it is demagoguery to contend that "money is the root of all evil." This demagoguery becomes pernicious in light of the greater evil of needlessly losing a life that could otherwise be saved, were we to dispense with arbitrary designations for what can or cannot be commodified. Free market economists concerned with addressing the scarcity of precious goods insist that a proscription against such a market on the grounds that "money corrupts" is simply a descriptor rather than a persuasive (and not very convincing) argument for or against. Perhaps it is time to look briefly at how a regulated market for organ trade would work, as well as how it does look in the one place in the world where such a market is legal: Iran.

THE UNIQUE CASE OF IRAN

In 1988 Iran implemented a program to allow for monetary compensation for living, unrelated donor renal transplantation. A decade later the Iranian government boasted that the country had solved its organ shortage supply problem.[41] While a completely accurate picture is obscured by our inability to obtain unfettered access to information about Iran's medical system, the general sense is that Iranians themselves are in support of such a system and that it has saved the Ministry of Health, now less burdened by expenditures on dialysis, substantial amounts of money.[42] Today, Iran is the only country in the world in which selling one's kidney for profit is legal. In order to minimize "medical tourism," keep the market safely regulated, and attend first and foremost to the needs of Iranian citizens, it is essentially an Iranian-only system:

kidneys procured from living non-family members can come from Iranian nationals only, and non-Iranians can participate in the system only if they are brought in for the benefit of an Iranian.[43]

Despite this somewhat limited sample size, the Iranian experience does provide an instance by which we can speculate as to how a real market for organ trade might work for both donors and recipients. Like many who favor an organ-for-market trade, Iran's is a highly regulated system. Donors are not matched with recipients via a series of individual contracts binding vendor to buyer. Rather, candidates for transplantation pay the donor, but the amount is always supplemented both by government subsidies and, depending on the financial abilities of the recipient, by contributions from nongovernmental organizations.[44] Together these three funding sources are enough to cover the donor's payment and the cost of the operation. Every transaction is overseen by a governmental agency.

While having multiple funding sources does imply some regional variation in pricing, the system also has the advantage of being comprehensive and able to address flexibly the needs of Iranian citizens with different financial strains and capabilities. In theory such government oversight also implies a fluid system of exchange in which there is an ongoing assessment of fair value in real time. In other words, and especially in light of the help provided by governmental subsidies and NGO donations, the market can correct for over- and underpricing when it needs to do so.

In Iran the whole process is facilitated by the existence of *Anjoman*, or the nonprofit living transplantation advocacy organizations that arrange for matches between donors and recipients. Sigrid Fry-Revere, president and co-founder of the American Living Organ Donor Network (ALODN), went through the long process of being approved to travel to Iran in order to investigate its government's claim to have solved the shortage problem through the creation of a market. She found that the *Anjoman* are the personnel designated to solve donors' long-term financial problems and make sure donors and their families are fully informed about every aspect of the transplantation process.[45]

While (as she admits) her exposure to the *Anjoman* was filtered through the Iranian government, Fry-Revere nevertheless witnessed a number of occasions on which these advocates went the extra mile to find a suitable match and made sure the distinctive needs of particular populations, such as the impoverished, were specially addressed. The good of the country, in terms of reputation and best medical practices, is preserved through the work of the *Anjoman*.[46] In Fry-Revere's estimation, this is how Iran incorporates the fundamental libertarian principle of affording the greatest number of options within the context of sensible regulations to ensure that vulnerable individuals are protected and that the commodification of organs does not come too easily. Before an unrelated and paid living donation is allowed, aggressive efforts are made to find a suitable organ from cadavers, from donors from within the family, or from altruistic donors.[47]

Despite the existence of a market for organ trade, paid living donation in Iran is seen as a last resort. Because, culturally, in Islamic societies shame is so often associated with individuals or families that persist in debt, every effort is made to attend to the long-term financial interests of the donors.[48] The going rate of a kidney is heavily monitored by the government so as to alleviate burdens carried by the donor, on the one hand, and to reach a reasonable market equilibrium, on the other. In the long term this helps to give credibility to donation as a viable alternative to dialysis.

There is another reason for this heavy hand. Unlike in the United States, where living donors welcome acknowledgment for their sacrifice, under the contractual arrangement brokered by the *Anjoman* donors mostly wish to remain anonymous because of the social stigma that arises from financial need. As Fry-Revere observes:

> Despite their awareness that they had done an honorable deed, they saw having sold a kidney as proof that they had fallen on hard times. Understandably, most people, whether kidney sellers or not, aren't in a rush to share their misfortunes with their neighbors, friends, or sometimes even their families. Sadly, people like Morad, who didn't donate out of financial desperation, were caught up in the stigma that all kidney donors are kidney sellers, and that only drug addicts or people who are otherwise failures in life sell their kidneys. . . . Dr. Malakoutian told us the medical community and the *Anjomans* in Tehran tried to arrange donor-appreciation events, even advertising them on television, but those efforts were a total bust.[49]

Clearly, a contrast can be drawn between the non-anonymous nature of living donation in places where sacrifice is not monetarily compensated and non-anonymous donation in places where donors prefer a business-like transaction in which they receive money.

While it may be tempting to conclude that it is the exchange of money that causes the undesirable stigma for donors, Fry-Revere, upon deeper investigation, believes that the problem is just the opposite: the organ market is still too anomalous and culturally conspicuous for it to have yet gained normative acceptance.[50] Still, while it might be a problem that in Iran at the moment kidney sellers motivated by the prospect of getting out of debt exist alongside others motivated by doing good, overall buy-in to the notion that one can help someone else while *simultaneously* helping oneself is, Fry-Revere believes, a sentiment on the rise.

Fry-Revere references a donor named Arman she interviewed at Hashem-inejad Hospital, who stressed that "donating a kidney is better than getting a government handout or going on government assistance, and maybe even borrowing money from family and friends."[51] In another example Fry-Revere describes a donor who invokes the Koran as support for the notion that it is a virtue to help oneself by helping others. The point is subtle: the tension one might observe between acting from altruistic and selfless motives is of a conditional nature. Initially, because of the way in which social stigmas wield widespread influence, it may be easy to draw an obvious contrast between those whose actions spring from other-regard and those who seem forced into other-regarding scenarios in order to attend to a more immediate and base ambition (such as delivering oneself from debt). However, it is possible for self-regarding and other-regarding motives to be integrated into the same social act. Once this happens enough times, it becomes a more powerful, stable practice than either of its two alternatives. This, in essence, captures the appeal of the Iranian system, according to Fry-Revere: the *Anjomans* see the most important component of their job as advocating equitably and compassionately on behalf of both donors and recipients to achieve outcomes that will lead to an enduring equilibrium.

Sigrid Fry-Revere concludes that a system built around this confluence of incentives provides a hopeful trajectory for the Iranian experiment. While it cannot be denied that money remains a prominent motivator for donors, the Iranian market has evolved since its inception over twenty-five years ago in at least a couple of critical ways:

> First, as the backlog of people needing kidneys diminished and the system developed a surplus of potential donors, the *Anjomans* and medical staffs became more selective about the people they chose as donors. Their selec-tivity was not limited to medical factors, such as eliminating drug users, but expanded to include social factors, such as picking donors whose lives could be changed in positive ways, financially or otherwise. Second, as a

surplus of donors developed, the price dropped, thus creating an atmosphere in conjunction with the aforementioned selectivity where helping individual donors with financial and psychological counseling began to take on new significance.[52]

Market efficiency leads to both the best pragmatic and the best moral outcomes. Such a conclusion is consistent with the assessments of Mark Cherry, James Stacey Taylor, and others, for whom the market is not only the most efficient means of closing the organ shortage gap but also a way of redressing ethical concerns of safety and exploitation—though perhaps not in the way one would have expected. With the help of the *Anjomans*, the Iranian system addresses the needs of donors and recipients and improves the morale of the entire transplant community.

A LEGAL, REGULATED MARKET FOR ORGAN TRADE

Proponents of legalizing the sale of organs believe there is much to learn from the case of Iran. Even if we remain skeptical about the claim that in Iran the shortage gap has been virtually solved because of the creation of a legal market for organ trade, maybe we could split the difference and assume that it largely has done so. How much better off we'd be, proponents surmise, by trying the experiment for a well-regulated market in the light of day, in an open society, under conditions of the best regulation. How would such a system work?

For starters, the system would not be one in which seller and buyer were left to their own devices to negotiate price and terms of sale. One of the most vocal proponents for legalization, transplant surgeon Dr. Arthur Matas, lays out in broad strokes the key guiding principles of a "regulated" system: it would be one in which a "fixed price is paid to the vendor (by the government or a government approved agency); the kidney is allocated by a predefined algorithm similar to that used for deceased donors (and everyone on the waiting list has opportunity to receive a vendor kidney); criteria are defined for vendor evaluation, acceptance and follow-up; and safeguards are adequate for vendor protection."[53] Such a system would provide safeguards against exploitation on either end by ensuring that organs didn't simply flow from the most desperate to the highest bidder; transactions would not be susceptible to being mediated by a corrupt broker.

A properly regulated system would avail itself of up-to-date means for screening donors to make sure they are healthy, and it would provide for consistent post-op checkups. These are features missing in a black or unregulated market. Participation would also be totally voluntary. No one would ever be coerced into donating. Recruitment would arguably place *less* pressure on prospective donors than in, for example, "opt-out" countries, in which cadaveric donation occurs by matter of course unless otherwise specified and where often at major gatherings (such as a fútbol match) a government-sponsored advertisement preaches to a captive audience about the virtues of remaining on the registry. There could be minimum-age restrictions, laws to make sure that discrimination against particular groups does not take place (as are currently on the books in cases of directed donation), and advantaging of natural or naturalized citizens over foreigners, depending on the political will of the nation.

This is all to say that in a regulated system, all logistics could be transparently handled by governmental agencies or representatives hired from the private sector that are best equipped to do so. The system would entail opportunities for evaluation and recalibration to make it better on an ongoing basis. It would allow for thorough scrutiny of vendors and make provisions for longitudinal studies of long-term health effects of donation. Finally, it would invite a range of voices to contribute to discussions about what reflects the most appropriate and reasonable amount for a lump-sum payment. As Cherry notes, there would also be a communal aspect to the creation of such a market:

> Rather than eroding a sense of community, the market may enhance and draw together moral communities, opening significant opportunities for developing personal relationships and for providing for the fundamental needs of others. Expressions of altruism may exist side by side with for-profit markets in human organs. For example, if it is altruism for a parent to give a kidney to a child to save his life, it is similarly altruistic for a parent to sell a kidney to pay for a lifesaving operation. Forbidding a market in human organs restricts persons from joining together with others to pool financial resources to purchase organs for the impecunious. It prevents altruistic donation of organs to nonprofit groups, who could then sell such parts to raise funds to purchase food, shelter, or health care for the poor. A market may open considerable opportunities for the expression of altruistic

sentiments, for building a sense of solidarity and community, as well as for charitably providing for the fundamental needs of others.[54]

Just as the *Anjomans* in Iran see themselves as the glue forging bonds between populations of society with different needs, the various stakeholders and brokers in an ideally regulated market would, by virtue of operating under assumptions of transparency and community-building, take on the role of a compassionate facilitator.

The "third-party" aspect of a solution based on a legal market is key. Cherry and other proponents suggest the introduction of vouchers as a way of providing protections for all of the relevant parties. Vouchers could function as a healthcare benefit provided by the state—for example, as part of Medicare or as a specified extension of Medicaid in which tax dollars lead to resources for the poor.[55] We have already determined as a society that dialysis is worth paying for as part of Medicare. Why could not a similar determination be made in the case of transplantations, which would over time save the system money? With a transparently visible middleman, one that could either be assigned by the government (as is the case of Iran) or come from the private sector, it is feasible within the context of a market to divorce the *procurement* of organs from their *allocation*. Donors could be paid in order to build up a bank of available organs, but we could still continue to rely on organizations like UNOS to set responsibly the criteria for who is eligible to be a recipient and with what priority level.

Regardless of where a price is set, any proposal of payment for a living donor will have an impact on and be perceived differently by those who exist in different financial situations.[56] In a regulated for-pay market, however, the government could specify the circumstances under which a third party could kick in an additional amount to neutralize this difference of socioeconomic circumstances. Donors would receive the same amount for their donation, but the amount a recipient would pay could fluctuate within an acceptable but revisable range, depending on his or her ability to pay. There is no reason a market *has* to be blind to demographical difference, in other words.

Such flexibility underscores Cherry's point about how a market can be conducive to communal objectives. If the creation of a market for organ trade can be made to be consistent with the same underlying principles in all of healthcare policy whereby we achieve, as a society, equitable distribution of scarce resources but remain sensitive to vulnerable populations, then there is nothing about the procurement of organs from paid living donors that should be resistant to addressing the disparate needs of our populace as a whole. Conversely, if our overall system is unjust, then so will be our means of procuring organs from living donors. The point is that there is no reason to think that procurement in a regulated system won't stand or fall with the system overall.

In sum, a responsibly implemented regulated market can have the flexibility to correct for injustice. Proponents do not deny that concerns about exploitation, equitable distribution of resources, safety, or the effect on vulnerable populations are real. But proponents are also quick to point out that the issue of addressing the organ shortage crisis is equally real and not a hypothetical debate about the nature of how virtuous intention can become corrupted. Human lives hang in the balance, and we need at all times to keep in the forefront of our mind those desperate parents who, if pressed, would go to any length to save their child in need of a lifesaving organ. While going out of their way to acknowledge ethical misgivings about the sale of organs, in the final analysis proponents for legalization nevertheless insist that it is a utilitarian and practical issue that should be considered first and foremost. They believe we ought to adopt the policy that will save the most lives, period.

NOTES

1. US Public Law 98–507, *National Organ Transplant Act* (NOTA) 98, Statute 2339 (1984).

2. Pope John Paul II, *Evangelium Vitae* no. 86, March 25, 1995. For the full text of the encyclical, see: http://w2.vatican.va/content/john-paul-ii/en/encyclicals /documents/hf_jp-ii_enc_25031995_evangelium-vitae.html.

3. One of the biggest myths surrounding organ donation is that the world's major religions do not lend support to the practice. For example, while Judaism and Islamism presume deference to burying the body whole, in both traditions it is also held that "necessity overrides prohibition." The website of the Halachic Organ Donor Society (HODS) offers a nice account from within the resources of Rabbinic Judaism of why Jews should advocate for organ donation. See https://www.hods.org/.

4. See Joel Feinberg, "Non-Coercive Exploitation," in *Paternalism*, ed. R. Sartorious (Minneapolis: University of Minnesota Press, 1983), 210; Samuel Rippon, "Imposing Options on People in Poverty: The Harm of a Live Donor Market," *Journal of Medical Ethics* 40 (2014): 145–48; and S. M. Rothman and D. J. Rothman, "The Hidden Cost of Organ Sale," *American Journal of Transplantation* 6, no. 7 (2006): 1524–28.

5. Kieran Healy, *Last Best Gifts: Altruism and the Market for Human Blood and Organs* (Chicago: University of Chicago Press, 2006), 118.

6. Mark J. Cherry, *Kidney for Sale by Owner: Human Organs, Transplantation, and the Market* (Washington, DC: Georgetown University Press, 2005), ix.

7. Ibid., 95.

8. Arthur J. Matas, "Why We Should Develop a Regulated System of Kidney Sales: A Call for Action!," *Clinical Journal of the American Society of Nephrology* 1 (2006): 1131.

9. Robert Kuttner, *Everything for Sale: The Virtues and Limits of Markets* (Chicago: University of Chicago Press, 1999), 64.

10. Abimereki D Muzaale et al., "Risk of End-Stage Renal Disease Following Live Kidney Donation," *Journal of the American Medical Association* 311, no. 6 (2013): 579–86. Muzaale and his colleagues compare the risk of end-stage renal disease among kidney donors with the risk among a comparably healthy cohort of non-donors. Because donors come from the healthiest population of individuals in society, it is hard to determine whether they are putting themselves at additional risk by donating. In one of the first longitudinal studies inquiring into whether there is such a correlation, the authors conclude that kidney donors have a somewhat higher estimated risk of developing ESRD throughout their lifetimes (90 per 10,000) compared to similarly healthy individuals who did not donate (14 per 10,000), but still a much lower risk than the general population (326 per 10,000).

11. Centers for Disease Control and Prevention, *National Diabetes Fact Sheet 2011* (Atlanta, GA: Centers for Disease Control and Prevention, US Department of Health and Human Services, 2011). See http://www.cdc.gov/diabetes/pubs/pdf/ndfs_2011 .pdf. As explained on the CDC fact sheet, type 2 diabetes was previously called non-insulin-dependent diabetes mellitus (NIDDM) or adult-onset diabetes. In adults, type 2 diabetes accounts for about 95 percent of newly diagnosed cases of diabetes. Like type 1 diabetes, type 2 usually presents as insulin resistance: as the need for insulin rises, the pancreas gradually loses its ability to produce it. Type 2 diabetes is at present associated with older age, obesity, family history of diabetes, history of gestational diabetes, impaired glucose metabolism, physical inactivity, and race/ethnicity, but not kidney donation.

12. A good example of this occurs in the field of dermatology, where private practices often consist of one large office with a series of examination rooms that wrap around to connect to two separate waiting rooms: one room over-packed with patients afflicted with psoriasis, acne, skin cancers, and so forth, and the other spa-like, holding those awaiting cosmetic procedures like Botox and face-lifts. See an example of such a practice in Chico, California, as reported in the *New York Times*: http://www.nytimes.com/2008/07/28/us/28beauty.html?_r=0.

13. Alexander Berger, "Why Selling Kidneys Should Be Legal," *New York Times*, December 5, 2011, http://www.nytimes.com/2011/12/06/opinion/why-selling-kidneys -should-be-legal.html?_r=0.

14. Amy Friedman, "Payment for Living Organ Donation Should Be Legalised," *British Medical Journal* 333 (2006): 746–48: http://www.ncbi.nlm.nih.gov/pmc /articles/PMC1592395/.

15. Ibid.

16. Cherry, *Kidney for Sale by Owner*, 31.

17. Michael Walzer, *Spheres of Justice: A Defense of Pluralism and Equality* (New York: Basic, 1983), 120.

18. Joel Feinberg, *Harms to Self* (New York: Oxford University Press, 1986), 252, discussed in Cherry, *Kidney for Sale by Owner*, 90.

19. Madhav Goyal et al., "Economic and Health Consequences of Selling a Kidney in India," *Journal of the American Medical Association* 288, no. 13 (2002): 1589–93.

20. Robert M. Veatch and Lainie F. Ross, *Transplantation Ethics*, 2nd ed. (Washington, DC: Georgetown University Press, 2015), 174, 176. Cherry, *Kidney for Sale by Owner*, 90.

21. Cherry, *Kidney for Sale by Owner*, 91.

22. Ibid.

23. Veatch and Ross, *Transplantation Ethics*, 176.

24. Margaret Jane Radin, *Contested Commodities* (Cambridge, MA: Harvard University Press, 1996), 142.

25. Ibid.

26. Ibid.

27. This is, unfortunately, not a hypothetical. In the not-that-uncommon case of fragile or unhealthy babies, buyers and sellers in the business of surrogacy often hire lawyers to protect their financial interests and shield themselves from liability, too often with insufficient regard for the infant life that hangs in the balance. For one such depressing example from 2012 in the state of Connecticut, see: http://www.cnn.com/2013/03/04/health/surrogacy-kelley-legal-battle.

28. For a discussion of this nation's frenzied bid to make conception and a successful birth urgent priorities in which to invest, see Paul Lauritzen, *Pursuing Parenthood: Ethical Issues in Assisted Reproduction* (Bloomington: University of Indiana Press, 2000).

29. See, for example, Veatch and Ross, *Transplantation Ethics,* 334.

30. Sally Satel, "Desperately Seeking a Kidney," *New York Times Magazine*, December 16, 2007, http://www.nytimes.com/2007/12/16/magazine/16kidney-t.html ?_r=0. See more on "coerced altruism" in Cherry, *Kidney for Sale by Owner*, 76, 94.

31. Renée Fox and Judith P. Swazey, *Spare Parts: Organ Replacement in American Society* (Oxford: Oxford University Press, 1992), 40. Satel quotes from Fox and Swazey in "Desperately Seeking a Kidney."

32. Satel, "Desperately Seeking a Kidney."

33. Ibid.

34. This was stated in episode 2 of *Free to Exchange*, the series broadcasted by a Texas Christian University–sponsored libertarian think tank (with host Ben Powell and guests James Stacey Taylor and Gilbert Berdine), https://www.youtube.com/watch?v=dzZla4KSBPM&feature=youtu.be.

35. Ibid.

36. Radin, *Contested Commodities*, 5,

37. James Stacey Taylor, "Libertarian Philosophy: Black Market—Should You Be Allowed to Sell Your Kidneys?" YouTube video posted by Learn Liberty, November 21, 2011. See https://www.youtube.com/watch?v=_--FhEk-pLw.

38. In America, too, we sadly have a precedent for exploitation at the behest of profiting middlemen who avail themselves of a black market in organ trade. A notable recent example is the Levy Izhak Rosenbaum case in 2009, which resulted in a number of arrests in New Jersey on charges of corruption, money laundering, and the bribery of municipal officials. Rosenbaum assisted both vendors and recipients of organs by fabricating stories to manipulate hospital physicians into believing paid donors were friends and family. In 2011 he confessed in federal court to brokering three illicit kidney transplants in exchange for payments of between $120,000 and $150,000, a crime for which he was sentenced to two and half years. Three New Jersey mayors and five rabbis were among those arrested. See Veatch and Ross, *Transplantation Ethics*, 172–73, 176.

39. Friedman, "Payment for Living Organ Donation," 747.

40. Sigrid Fry-Revere, *The Kidney Sellers: A Journey of Discovery in Iran* (Durham, NC: Carolina Academic Press, 2014), 7.

41. For a succinct explanation of the Iranian system, see Veatch and Ross, *Transplantation Ethics*, 172. For an evaluation of the assertion by the Iranian government to have eliminated its organ shortage gap in 1999, see Benjamin E. Hippen, "Organ Sales and Moral Travails: Lessons from the Living Kidney Vendor Program in Iran," *Cato Policy Analysis Series* (2008): 614.

42. Veatch and Ross, *Transplantation Ethics*, 173.

43. Ibid.

44. Ibid.

45. Fry-Revere, *Kidney Sellers*, 123.

46. Ibid., 51.

47. Ibid., 57.

48. For a source that refutes this claim, see Javaad Zargooshi, "Iranian Kidney Donors: Motivations and Relations with Recipients," *Journal of Urology* 165 (2001): 386–92. Zargooshi reports on the shame that Iranians who sell their kidneys claim to feel post-donation. Fry-Revere is herself ambivalent about the extent to which the Iranian system ultimately makes the standard of living better for donors and their families. See Fry-Revere, *Kidney Sellers*, 87.

49. Fry-Revere, *Kidney Sellers*, 88–89.

50. Ibid., 89.

51. Ibid., 90.

52. Ibid., 157.

53. Arthur J. Matas, "The Case for Living Kidney Sales: Rationale, Objections, and Concerns," *American Journal of Transplantation* 4 (2004): 2008.

54. Cherry, *Kidney for Sale by Owner*, 102.

55. Ibid., 77.

56. Veatch and Ross, *Transplantation Ethics*, 179.

2

Ethical Concerns with Legalizing
the Sale of Organs

THE UTILITY OF UTILITY

Those in favor of legalizing the sale of organs through the creation of a market believe that doing so would not only optimize our prospects for closing the gap between organs in demand and willing donors, but also that it would do so in an ethically sound manner, in part by providing an alternative to the black market that imperils public safety and exploits both donors and recipients. The first of these two claims, that a market for organ trade reduces the shortage gap, will be considered in chapter 3. But first, the second claim about exploitation must be scrutinized by looking more closely at proponents' conviction that a legal and transparent market makes the overall environment for organ trade more equitable and safer for sellers and buyers while violating no maxim against commodification of a sacred good.

On the basis of the earlier discussion, we can grant that most proponents are responsibly aware of the risk of taking unacceptable shortcuts in incentivizing living donors to sacrifice an organ. However, these proponents additionally insist that the public is vulnerable to exploitation or otherwise endangered only when an organ receives a price tag in the context of the black market. Is this so? For example, what, if any, are the ethical concerns inherent in a clean, regulated market created to reduce society's dependence on dialysis and to give those suffering from end-stage renal disease a new lease on life with a transplanted kidney?

In this chapter, I now take up this question by delving into three ethical objections that have traditionally been leveled against the legalization of the sale of organs: (1) that the practice exploits the donor, particularly the impoverished one; (2) that the practice violates basic tenets of best medical practices, putting the public's health at risk; and (3) that the practice, by subjecting a good normally not for sale to market forces, disregards social mores customarily associated with the giving act. While these objections are conceptually distinct from the pragmatic question of whether legalizing the sale of organs will reduce the organ shortage per se, all three do relate to the issue. Particularly when taking public perception into account, ethics and utility have a lot to do with one another.

Organ transplantation involves a major surgery, and on a rare occasion something will go wrong and a healthy, willing donor unexpectedly becomes sick or even dies while attempting to make a sacrifice for a recipient in need. Typically this leads to the practice of organ donation being scrutinized anew by the press. Any discovery of ethical breaches that could have been avoided is likely to erode the public's already tentative trust in the practice of organ donation and transplantation. For this reason, it is not just for the sake of doing the right thing that transplantations are undertaken cautiously and in a manner that provides the maximum amount of protection for the donor. As in most instances of medical ethics, a perception problem arises because of an underlying real problem. Thus, if we are going to legalize the sale of bodily organs, we had better think through in advance how the promise of a monetary reward will alter the behavior of the rewarded.

This is not to say that there aren't good reasons to build a robust program of living donation. We have already noted that transitioning from dialysis to transplantation carries significant advantages for both the patient and society. Living donation is less expensive and allows the recipient to no longer merely survive by means of getting to and from scheduled infusions around which every week is planned. The recipient can circle back into the workforce and live each day with renewed opportunity. On medical grounds, if posed with a choice between the options of cadaveric and living donation, moreover, the latter is preferable: there is less ischemic time for the transplanted organ, which means that the duration at which the kidney (or partial liver lobe) to be transplanted must remain at body temperature is shorter, minimizing susceptibility to degeneration after blood supply has been cut off. This keeps the organ(s) viable longer. In living donation, surgeries are performed in adjacent operating rooms, so no planes or helicopters are required to transport the organ from one place to another. In every other aspect of transplantation, living donation allows time and flexibility around which to plan and coordinate the two procedures.

All of this suggests that the proponents of legalization are correct to complain that moralism, or adherence to ethical principles for their own sake, is not a good enough reason to stick to the old system of relying on voluntary donations only. Because of everything at stake, it is important to determine how serious the concerns actually are about safety, exploitation, and commodification, as well as examine any empirical data we have at our disposal with which to come to an informed conclusion.

We know something about the effects of policies for legalizing the sale of organs from studies and investigative exposés conducted in countries where the practice was once legal or, in the case of Iran, still is legal. India, where selling organs was prevalent until it became illegal in 1994—though it is still occurring, on the black market—is the part of the world from which we have the best available information. But we also know something about the effects of creating a market for organ trade from observations in the Philippines, where selling organs was legal until 2008, and China, where the practice became illegal in 2010 after Human Rights Watch uncovered evidence that Falun Gong prisoners were being executed to free up their kidneys for consumption in the marketplace.[1] If selling organs were to become legal in the United States, it would presumably occur under the transparency enjoyed in a free society. That said, what occurred in China was not the result of black market abuse. Rather, it was state-sanctioned murder under the watchful eye of a government interested only in solving a problem in a practical way. The point here is that the introduction of money can change human behavior, possibly beyond a threshold of moral acceptability.

Whereas the example of executing prisoners for their organs is extreme and should be counted as a grotesquely criminal act, it is not hard to imagine how the prospect of profiting from the sale of organs ethically complicates policy. What if, as a result of legalizing the sale of organs, it turned out that a kidney became a relatively expensive item for purchase and individuals with transplanted organs were predominantly wealthy whereas their paid donors were predominantly impoverished? We have to ask if this is the kind of society we want to create, even if the organ shortage problem were to improve. It is no stretch of the imagination to speculate that a legal organ trade would feed into the already growing disparity between the so-called 1 percent and everyone else. A purchased organ could become an additional symbol of privilege among society's elite. In capitalistic societies the rich have, and are expected to have, things that most others lack. If organs can be bought, there is no reason to think they won't become another luxury item available to the few. This issue of disparity, moreover, is compounded by the difficulty of assuring informed consent among prospective donors in dire financial need. Legalizing the sale of organs introduces the prospect of protecting populations ripe for exploitation against the consequences of their own decision-making.

Nor is it hard to imagine how public safety could become imperiled by introducing a financial incentive that induces prospective donors to falsify their social and medical histories and hide factors that might otherwise exclude them from being eligible to donate. Much of this concern, it is true, is allayed by the battery of clinical tests currently being performed on prospective donors to validate their eligibility. These tests are both expensive and not completely fail-safe, however. A system that must be able to ferret out medically appropriate donors from among a pool now enlarged because of the prospect of financial reward could lead to errors resulting in the transmission of a disease in the transplantation process. More likely it will result in scenarios in which recipients must change their plans abruptly when a problem is discovered late in the process. In cases where the new organ is coming from a specific donor, the recipient will have stopped looking for other donors and so will have little time with which to begin anew the search to find a suitable match.

There is finally the conceptually murky yet critically important concept of commodification. Is there some sacred or ineffable quality inherent in bodily organs that precludes them from being exchanged in the open market? One can point to both theological and secular justifications for thinking so. From a theological perspective, there is something disturbing about placing a price tag on a nonregenerative body part over which only the divine is supposed to have dominion.[2] According to the sanctity of life doctrine, humans are the exemplification of God's prized creatures, and we do not have a "blank check" to do to our bodies whatever we choose.[3]

In addition to theological arguments against commodification, critics worry that subjecting some goods to the marketplace will lead to a devaluing of relations between the buyers and sellers of such goods. This broader secular objection is more subtle and more complicated to defend than its theological counterpart as, unlike sectarian arguments based on faith, it has pretensions of a pluralistic appeal to shared notions of fellowship and goodwill. Does commodification entail an erosion of trust between two parties whose capacity to bond with one another is weakened with the introduction of financial incentives? If love for neighbor wanes when it is no longer the only avenue for giving to the neighbor in need, then love's disappearance from society, aside from the impact that the gift normally brings about, also represents a legitimate area for ethical reflection. Let us now turn to the issues of exploitation, safety, and commodification.

SELLING ORGANS AND THE IMPOVERISHED

There are reasons of economy and compassion for why we would want to transition from a society that addresses kidney failure by relying mostly on dialysis to one that incorporates and favors transplantations. Such a shift would not only be a cheaper option over the long run; it would also give the ailing a new lease on life. These benefits, however, must be weighed against potential costs that society might bear for facilitating such a transition. If we accept the argument put forth by Robert Veatch and others, that, given that we have failed them institutionally in other respects we should as a last resort give poor individuals the option of selling their kidneys to alleviate some of their financial burdens—assuming the kidneys are valued at a sufficiently high price so as both to attract donors and adequately compensate them for their sacrifice—the next question we must ask is: Who are the likely donors and recipients in such an arrangement? Some estimates place the cost of a kidney at roughly $150,000.[4] Who is likely to be most persuaded into receiving such a large financial windfall? And who will be able to pay this amount?[5]

These questions beckon the sort of reflection raised by science fiction author Ursula Le Guin, as described in her short story "The Ones Who Walk Away from Omelas."[6] Le Guin's narrative depicts an annual seasonal festival in a utopian village where the village's residents lead a blissful existence characterized by plentitude, love, playfulness, and egalitarianism. However, for reasons that are vague and not really important, it becomes clear that this happiness is entirely dependent on the horrendous suffering of one innocent child who is perpetually kept locked and miserable in a dark, soiled dungeon, a fact that ritually becomes known to all once they are old enough to be told the truth. Upon learning of the sacrificial child's ordeal, almost everyone is naturally disgusted; most, however, are convinced to reevaluate this reaction in short order. Le Guin explains the reasoning through the voice of her narrator: "To exchange all the goodness and grace of every life in Omelas for that single, small improvement: to throw away the happiness of thousands for the chance of the happiness of one: that would be to let guilt within the walls indeed."[7] The citizenry are described as intelligent and compassionate, and it is clear that everyone knows what is at stake. While most succumb to the concession of abiding the unjust fate of one child, there is a small minority who can't live with the revealed cost of their enjoyed bliss. These are the ones who "walk away" from Omelas. Silent and in disbelief, they travel to a destination not revealed to the reader but that Le Guin implies is not idyllic like Omelas and is a place too strange even to be imagined.

To Le Guin's credit, the decision to stay in or walk away is presented as an interesting and difficult one and a legitimate analog to the kinds of decisions that societies must collectively make when there is no perfect solution. Anyone who retains status as an inhabitant of Omelas, acquiescing to the choice that must be made in order to hold on to a blissful existence, has ample intellectual cover for doing so. Nevertheless, we are meant to acknowledge the minority, for whom the ethical cost is too high to stay behind. Returning to the dilemma at hand, a similar question arises: Would we choose to live in a society in which the organ shortage problem could be eliminated if it meant using the bodies of the impoverished as "spare parts" for the rich?[8] There is surely a point at which we have to concede that solving the organ shortage problem is not worth the collateral damage that such incentivizing policies would bring. However undignified it is that society allows victims of serious renal disease to "wait with dignity for the organ that never comes," it is even less dignified to solve the problem on the backs of the needy in a manner that overtly favors the resource-rich.

In anticipation of this concern, proponents propose a regulated market for the pricing of organs that is in alignment with both what most recipients could afford and what donors should reasonably receive (see chap. 1). They argue for the existence of an achievable point of equilibrium at which it is plausible to imagine that a financial reward is consistent with, and does not undermine, the altruistic spirit with which a donation is intended, thereby reducing the likelihood of producing one donor class in contrast to a different recipient class. The problem with this response, however, is that it cuts against the libertarian insight that it is the free market itself that naturally corrects for misplacement of value and resolves problems of supply and demand. Regulate the market too much and we will not attract a sufficient number of healthy, appropriate donors to step forward (and may actively prevent the sort of redistribution of wealth that Veatch counts as an economic benefit to the creation of a market for body parts). This leads to a catch-22: regulating a legal market potentially could be discriminatory, but not regulating it makes the poor even more susceptible to exploitation. Such discrimination, furthermore, places questionable constraints on whoever is deemed to be a suitable donor. If Veatch is right, should not the poor everywhere have equal access to the opportunities to better their lot by becoming paid donors?

Sheila Rothman and David Rothman express this tension poignantly:

> Some proponents would restrict the sale to U.S. citizens, but the limitation seems neither logical nor appropriate. Why penalize green card holders or long-term residents? Or for that matter, tourists or illegal immigrants? Since the goal is to maximize the number of organs since kidney sale ostensibly benefits the vendor, why exclude anyone? Why should not the poor of Bombay enjoy an option given to the poor of Appalachia? Why deprive a patient of a kidney because the seller must travel? The end result, however, might give new meaning to the lines of Emma Lazarus engraved on the Statue of Liberty: "Give me your tired, your poor . . . the wretched refuse of your teeming shore."[9]

It would seem that once we seriously propose legalizing a market for organ trade, we also, by way of natural course, lose control over how things will develop over time. Yet the alternative—a well-intended paternalism—is discriminatory, potentially xenophobic, and also, from the perspective of the market, less efficient. Moreover, regulation is hard to enforce. Such an experiment actually played out in the United States when it became legal to sell blood plasma and tissue for industrial and commercial purposes: a precipitous influx of our neighbors from the south interested in the opportunity ensued.[10]

For this reason Rothman and Rothman refer to "the myth of the regulated market" in which policies, designed to stave off some of the most predictable ethical misgivings associated with the sale of organs, are proposed without any real likelihood of their being implemented, lest the incentive-driven appeal of the market, which is what makes it an attractive option in the first place, lose any of its luster. So, while most proponents in free societies reject a public auction, within which the kidney goes to the highest bidder, in favor of distribution overseen by a UNOS-like organization (permitting individuals to sell but not buy organs), such compromises directly undermine the way in which a market is supposed to work. According to market assumptions, we are most likely to do something when we are well paid for it.[11] It is therefore hard to reap the benefits of the legalization of a market if one is not "all in." Half-measures that pay sellers but preclude the creation of buyers will turn out to be, if not inoperative, then at best inefficient:

Effectively regulated markets typically involve so-called "natural monopolies" wherein entry points can be effectively policed. (Think of electric power, telephone service and railroads.) By contrast, in kidney sale, with almost everyone eligible to enter the market, oversight will not be easily established or maintained. So too, as most students of regulated markets are quick to admit, change almost inevitably carries unintended consequences. Deregulate the market in energy trading and Enron scandals occur; deregulate the telephone market and the communications industry is transformed; deregulate the savings and loan business and corruption breaks out. Hence, the question must be asked: since practices may develop in ways that cannot be predicted or controlled, are we ready to live with a system that makes kidneys a commodity?[12]

The authors here raise an additional concern beyond whether we can trust individuals in desperate need to act in their own best interests if their rent is due and they need to put food on the table. There is legitimate concern about exploitation when such individuals are forced into participation in such a market, and also the fact that the market itself, once created, becomes its own monster.

We often do not know the macro-consequences of new opportunities in commerce before the trade of the new goods have been made legal. An example of this occurred in California in the early 2000s. The decision to deregulate the purchase of energy sources when the state's consumption needs unexpectedly spiked led to price gouging on the part of Texas oilmen, which in turn led Californians to vote via proposition for extremely unfavorable bonds that prioritized short-term access to cash so these needs could be met. In the long run, however, the decision, which seemed necessary at the time, thrust the state into a series of rolling brownouts and a budgetary crisis for years after.[13] It is conceivable that the legalization of the sale of kidneys, which would have to be priced high enough to attract enough willing donors, would, despite our best efforts, produce a market for the flow of a prized and scarce good leading directly from the poor to the rich and exponentially adding to already existing problems of disparity and class in ways that cannot be anticipated in advance.

We therefore have reason to regard with suspicion Veatch's well-intended allowance, sprung from a liberal perspective about procuring conditions of social justice, that selling organs represents an opportunity to reduce disparity between the classes. What begins in a free market as a voluntary enterprise can transform into a situation in which the worst off have the most reduced access to the good that the market was supposed to have made more plentiful, independent of the direction of any specific actor. As R. W. Evans notes, this should come as no surprise. The economics of organ transplantation is reflective of our medical system in general. Even after the passage of the Affordable Care Act, the "ability to pay is a condition of access that characterizes all of medical care in a health care delivery system such as ours. Transplantation is simply a specific example, more poignant only because of the immediacy of the life and death crisis."[14] Evans implies that to the extent that we move in the direction of a market, where adult sellers and buyers are free to make their own decisions, we move away from valuable social umbrellas such as Medicare, which are intended to make access more equitable.[15] This might not be the principal concern of specific individuals who remain preoccupied with their acute set of needs, but third parties are nevertheless inevitably affected.

One example of this effect is reported by anthropologist Lawrence Cohen, whose ethnographic research concludes that in places where kidney selling is prevalent, such as the Tamil countryside, "operable women [have become] vehicles for debt collateral."[16] Expanding on Cohen's findings, Deborah Satz points out that despite the fact that proponents of markets for organ sale are concerned with individual transactions within a given environment, those environments themselves are changed by the introduction of buying and selling. According to Satz, as Cohen's research suggests, "if kidney selling became widespread, a poor person who did *not* want to sell her kidney might find it harder to obtain loans."[17] Satz makes a similar point about child labor and other sorts of undercutting that occur when desperate individuals within shared environments allow themselves to be exploited because of conditions of ubiquitous desperation. "Ceteris paribus, the credit market allocates loans to people who can provide better collateral," as Satz writes. "If a kidney market exists, the total amount of collateral rises, which means that those without spare kidneys or those that refuse to sell them, will get fewer loans than before."[18] This is something that even in a monitored context is hard to regulate against, and it underscores the coercive effect on third parties when transactions are imagined in theory as occurring between only two parties.

More straightforwardly, it is also not clear that kidney selling presents a unique opportunity for the impoverished to lift themselves up out of dire financial straits or that it can be sustained on its own merits. The few empirical studies we have to test such a hypothesis have emerged from studying the case of India, where selling kidneys was legal until 1994. Madhav Goyal and colleagues demonstrate that the sale of kidneys by poor people in India not only did not lead to tangible benefit for the seller but, if anything, led to both a worsening of economic status and provided a false cover for middlemen who profited from the practice when it was legal.[19] Goyal's study was conducted in Chennai, a sizable city of over six million people in southern India, which had acquired the reputation of being a "kidney selling zone" by attracting individuals and families in debt. Almost all of the surveyed participants sought to sell their kidneys to get out of a debt in order to afford basic needs such as food and household expenses, rent, marriage expenses, and medical expenses.[20] Kidney sellers in this study did not report that they sought to "get rich quick"; rather, they entertained the option of selling an organ simply to continue subsisting at their same barely modest standard of living. Of the more than three hundred participants, forty-seven reported that a spouse had also sold a kidney.[21] Among all participants, the overall family income declined from $660 at the time of the nephrectomy to $420 by the time of the survey, while the percentage of participants below the poverty line increased from 54 percent to 71 percent.[22] Nearly 80 percent regretted their decision, indicating they would not recommend that others do as they had done. A great percentage reported receiving less than they thought they had been promised, and over three-quarters of the sampled participants complained they were still in debt after a few months. Commenting on the effect the legalization of selling kidneys has on the poor in developing countries such as India, where the practice of selling organs on the surface carries the most appeal, Goyal and his coauthors conclude that

> potential donors need to be protected from being exploited. At a minimum, protection might involve education about the likely outcomes of selling a kidney. Some have commented that rather than protecting poor people, authorization committees simply provide a cover for illegal cash-for-kidney deals. . . . [Moreover], a majority of donors were women. Given the often weak position of women in Indian society, the voluntary nature of some donations is questionable.[23]

Debt collectors, furthermore, became more aggressive in kidney-selling zones in the Chennai region, making the system of selling organs for cash a self-reinforcing phenomenon that worsened rather than ameliorated conditions of economic disparity and poverty.

One can't help but reject the notion that selling an organ represents a viable means to attaining upward social mobility. On the contrary, the worse off someone is at the start, the more susceptible he or she is to having even more limited options and less autonomy *after* selling an organ. This conclusion is further intensified in the case of marginalized individuals in society, such as women in India. "In addition to allocation concerns," writes J. Randall Boyer, "laissez faire systems tend to benefit sophisticated actors in the market at the expense of weaker, less sophisticated parties who hold much less bargaining power."[24] Thus, it is unfair in the first place that the poor might find themselves being forced into commerce not in their best interests and, secondarily, that they will suffer the additional injury of being taken advantage of by profiteers who further coerce them into inequitable arrangements. The right kind of regulation can go some distance toward mitigating these pernicious outcomes, but only by not earmarking the impoverished for financial betterment, which weakens Robert Veatch's claim from the other direction. Even if we manage to create a system that avoids this worst outcome, an expectation will still settle in the public mind that, to quote the political philosopher Peter Lawler, "your kidney might be understood as part of your net wealth."[25] Over time this will amount to a violation of one of the basic tenets of distributive justice: the poor would disproportionately come to supply kidneys for the rich, but, due to a lack of resources, they would by and large not be able to purchase them.[26] We are right back at the gates of Omelas.

Finally, there is the psychological question of the extent to which needy individuals, presented with the prospect of receiving a large sum of money overnight, are prone to act rashly in ways that are not in their best interests. Here the concern is that there is a threshold of reward beyond which any promise made to the recipient is intoxicatingly alluring. When they looked at risk-taking in investments and financial markets, psychologists Camelia Kuhnen and Brian Knutson discovered that anticipating certain sudden financial windfalls affects actor rationality in economic decision-making.[27] Using fMRI technology, Kuhnen and Knutson found that the nucleus accumbens shows heightened neural activity when subjects are presented with the prospect of securing significant financial betterment, even if such activity is risky. Selling a kidney could be packaged as one of the few "get-rich-quick" schemes theoretically available to anyone. As such, it could trigger the same sorts of addictive and harmful behaviors as playing the stock market. To counter that preventing donors from making their own decisions is prohibitively paternalistic is misleading. Given that the mechanisms these researchers describe are already under way when the mind is teased with the prospect of receiving a lump sum of money, the option to sell arguably becomes a form of entrapment. Under certain circumstances the promise of money becomes pervasively toxic to those who perceive themselves to be most in need of it. Kuhnen and Knutson's research shows that, from the perspective of the donor's experience, there is a qualitative difference between being modestly compensated for burdens one will endure in the transplantation process and receiving a significant sum of money beyond this compensatory amount. To paraphrase the psychologists who have studied the phenomenon, in the latter case all bets are off.

SELLING ORGANS AND PUBLIC SAFETY

The idea that desperate donors might be induced into acting contrary to their long-term interests leads to reflection over the safety of donors, recipients, and the society in which selling organs is legal. On June 2, 2011, a seventeen-year-old teenager in the Hunan Province of China sold his kidney in order to buy an iPad2. He reportedly received 20,000 yuan (the equivalent of just over $3,000), a sale that at the time was technically illegal in China even though a broker was nevertheless able to contact him over the Internet with relative ease. Quickly regretting his decision, by the time the parties who brokered the deal went on trial, the teen was in renal failure.[28]

While it bears mentioning that this episode occurred on the black market and is therefore not analogous to what would happen in a regulated, sanctioned context, the event does describe many prospective donors, who perceive themselves as desperate, and the safety ramifications of their decisions. Can such a correlation be defended? Again, it is useful to refer to Goyal's study, which was conducted following India's experiment with legalization. As he and his colleagues report, participants evaluated their health before their nephrectomies relative to afterward by using a standard 5-point scale (ranging from excellent to poor). Few reported no decline in health; nearly 40 percent reported a 1- to 2-point decline; and nearly 50 percent reported a 3- to 4-point decline. Approximately 50 percent noted persistent pain at the site of incision, while one-third complained of back pain.[29] According to the World Health Organization, in Iran 58 percent of donors experience poor health following nephrectomies, and more express regret over donating.[30]

The skeptic might be inclined to dismiss these as the findings in a developing country only. Were selling to become legal the United States, nephrectomies likely would continue to occur under the same sterile and safe conditions that they already are. It is possible, however, that as demand increases, so will the likelihood that normal protocols and safeguards would be placed under duress and lead to important conflicts of interest and unanticipated dangers to the safety of donors and recipients.

There is precedent in medical ethics for the need to protect people against themselves as well as to make sure that they are fully informed when undergoing any kind of risky procedure or operation. Recall that despite the moral good entailed in the gesture, there is no medical benefit to one who donates his or her kidney. By default this places the procedure or surgery in the "elective" category—that is, it is not required to save or even improve the health of the patient. As a rule of thumb, any elective surgery should carry less than a .5 percent risk of complication or death. Just as ophthalmologists who perform Lasik or Lasek are obligated to let their patients know if their corneas are too thin to meet the standard cautionary guideline—regardless of the degree to which those patients desire to be free of their glasses or contact lenses—so, too, are surgeons who perform nephrectomies required to explain thoroughly the procedure to prospective donors in such a way that fully informs them of the risks they face. The libertarian's conviction is that it is the individual alone who should have final say over the decision. However, in medical ethics the prerogative to put oneself at risk is never an unconditional trump card. As Randall Boyer argues, the health consequences "from selling body parts for desperately needed money may justify governmental restraint on individual liberty," because desperation may "drive a potential donor to focus too much on the benefit and fail to seek enough information about the risks, resulting in hasty decisions that do not account for potential future health costs."[31] Autonomy, then, is not the overriding principle in play here. There can be no human "right" to becoming a donor, whether paid or unpaid, because it would be disastrous to let a prospective donor intentionally incur a poor health risk, both for that donor himself and for all future donors (and recipients) poised to participate appropriately in the transplantation process.

Another sort of case can be made that legalizing the sale of organs is unsafe for recipients. While we now have sophisticated technologies by which to test the blood of donors to identify communicable diseases, cancers, and so forth from a donor who should be screened out, a revision to the donation system could lead to an increase in frenetic, impulsive decision-making and overstress a system initially designed to work within the normal assumptions of voluntary donation. On whose shoulders should the burden fall to ensure that potential donors tell the truth when physicians record their social histories?[32] In a cash-for-donation system, donors who seek remedies for pressing urgencies may not prioritize their unknown recipients' well-being. Thus, as Boyer notes, the cost of legalization entails the mental and physical consequences of the donor and the "costs for recipients as well, should donors seek to conceal disease or health conditions from procurement companies in order to bargain for higher prices" or be considered eligible for payment for their organs.[33]

In fact, safety concerns ultimately caused the sale of blood to become illegal in this country. Richard Titmuss called donors of blood for profit in the late 1960s "skid row suppliers," referring primarily to the prevalence of hepatitis in the blood supply in the United States when selling blood was legal; this was not the case in England and Wales, where blood could only be donated voluntarily.[34] Worse, argued Titmuss, commercial blood suppliers drove altruistic donors away: while such donors were not motivated by the prospect of being paid, they also did not want to be deprived of the reputation attendant to that of a good citizen who donates blood for his neighbor. Legalizing the sale of blood, in other words, led to a kind of adverse selection where blood donors disproportionately came from demographic categories least likely to be safe to donate. As a result of the attention Titmuss drew to the dangers of paid blood donors contaminating the blood supply, in 1973 the Department of Health, Education, and Welfare crafted a National Blood Policy that conceded that "commercial sources of blood and blood components for transfusion therapy has contributed to a significantly disproportionate incidence of hepatitis, since such blood is often collected from sectors of society in which transmissible hepatitis is more prevalent."[35] Since then the United States, like England and Wales, has had an all-volunteer system for the collection of blood.

While we should not conclude from this biographical note that making it illegal to sell blood is the only effective way to keep the blood supply free from contaminants, it does stand to reason that any system that involves incentives that increase the likelihood that one will lie on a medical questionnaire, designed and presented to keep the public safe, will not be an advantage to the public, even if such a system elicits a short-term increase in available blood.[36] Not only is this not in the public's overall interests, but just one publicized case of contaminated blood could do irreparable damage to the buy-in to blood donation over a long period of time. On the heels of the Institute of

Medicine's proclamation that blood ought not to be for sale because of this concern in 1973, the passage of NOTA in 1984 followed in kind. Better safe than sorry.

Today many safety concerns could be addressed in a market allowing for the sale of organs. The advancement of technology already allows for the possibility of efficient and accurate means of detecting eligible donors. We have, as a medicalized society, acquired enough experience with the transplantation process to be able to streamline the gathering of relevant information, regardless of whether or not the prospective donor is paid or unpaid. In light of this the critic may be prone to ask: Why, then, do we continue to proscribe the sale of organs if the objection is based on safety concerns?

The answer has to do with the power of incentives. While, given today's technological resource for conducting accurate tests, questionnaires are at most departure points for the acquisition of critical information, there is a valid "slippery slope" concern that warrants consideration, even when reliable checks and balances are at our disposal. The sale of organs introduces a conflict of interest between those responsible for procurement and those charged with ensuring the safety of the recipient. In a practical, if not theoretical, way it is difficult to guarantee that the process of obtaining willing, informed consent *and* truthful disclosure will not be influenced in the slightest by the immediacy and urgency that accompany financial incentives.

As the organ shortage problem becomes more pronounced, there will naturally be more pressure to rethink criteria for eligibility. We see this happening already, for example, with designated "expanded criteria" for procurement and with respect to acquiring organs from older donors (at present these are earmarked for older recipients only). As economists have often noted with regard to many goods for sale, markets by nature come to acquire an independence from the original purpose for which the goods being sold are put to use. This happens without any particular individual or group being responsible for effecting the change. Such an independence in the case of bodily organs, however, is dangerous if the buyer and the seller are led away from the third-party physicians or living donor advocates responsible for certifying that the interests of all are at all times being protected. The point, again, is a familiar one: hands-on regulation is the only remedy for guaranteeing safety. However, the more a market is regulated the less it is able to respond efficiently to demand and supply or to serve as an opportunity to entice new participants.

The conservative, cautionary best practices of ensuring safety are also not always in keeping with experiments to widen recruitment. While much can be regulatorily done to mitigate against this potential conflict of interest, the existence of the latter will always put added pressure on overseers trying to ensure the maintenance of the former. Even with sophisticated technology that enables us to screen carefully for blood-borne illness, the safest approach is still the one in which blood and organs are procured strictly through voluntary donation. Hence in 2013 the World Health Organization, in an attempt to dissuade countries from adopting policies that permitted the sale of blood or organs, published the following pronouncement: "Evidence shows significantly lower prevalence of transfusion-transmissible infections among voluntary non-remunerated donors than among other types of donors."[37]

COMMODIFICATION

The concerns about the exploitation of the impoverished and public safety are primarily tangible that result from the exchange of a precious good in an open market. The objection based on commodification is a little bit different, as it also raises the question about the spirit with which the referenced gift is exchanged. As Margaret Jane Radin notes:

> The ungainly word "commodification" denotes a particular social construction of things people value, their social construction as commodities. Commodification refers to the social process by which something comes to be apprehended as a commodity, as well as to the state of affairs once the process has taken place.[38]

According to this definition, commodities, or goods that are normally proffered as gifts but subsequently acquire a price tag, inherently affect more than just what they themselves concretely entail. This makes them susceptible to becoming *contested* goods because the process of subjecting normally unsellable items to the open market precipitates instances of personal and social conflict, particularly when the giver is deprived of connecting with a recipient. How a good can be worth more than its tangible value is perhaps a counterintuitive notion to grasp. Radin reflects on how this occurs in the case of human organs with a compelling thought experiment:

> Imagine the case of grief-stricken parents being asked to donate the heart of a brain-dead child to a newborn victim of a congenital heart disease in

a distant hospital. The parents are being asked to give up the symbolic integrity of their child and face immediately the brute fact of death. The act of donating the heart may be one of those distinctively human moments of terrible glory in which one gives up a significant aspect of oneself so that others may live and flourish. But now imagine the experience if the grieving parents know that the market price of the heart is $50,000. There seems to be a sense that the heroic moment now cannot be, either for them to experience or for us to observe, in respect and perhaps recognition. If the parents take the money, then the money is the reason for their actions; or at best, neither we nor they themselves will ever know that the money was not the reason for the action. But if they don't take the money, then their act can seem like transferring "their" $50,000 to the transplant recipient.[39]

The introduction of money comes at the cost of a precious social good: namely, the ability to aspire to and foster a certain identity as a civic-minded and socially conscious neighbor—if not a "hero" per se—who is free to act, and to be perceived as acting, out of the motive to offer help to one in need. The formation of this identity, as with the formation of all identities, depends on more than just individual volition. It also depends on social context. The conversion of a precious good into something that can be commodified critically affects this social context for everyone. This example refers to one possible instance of cadaveric donation, but the point can be generalized: the introduction of money in exchange for an organ, constituted as a regularly accepted practice, affects third parties beyond the donor (or donor's family) and recipient. Once something becomes monetized, it becomes monetized for everyone.

In *What Money Can't Buy*, Michael Sandel characterizes commodification similarly, as a process by which the introduction of monetary exchange changes a good from what it previously had been. Specifically, he sees it as a process whereby markets reduce different ways of valuing things to a singular dimension measured in money. This leads to the debasement of that good for both the giver and eventual possessor.[40] Such debasement can occur, for example, in the case of someone buying an academic degree or buying the friendship of another. When selling or buying these goods, one betrays his or her lack of understanding about what these goods in fact are, or to what their "internal" essence and function refers.[41]

There are other consequences to monetizing precious goods. Consider the example of our topic at hand. When body parts become acceptable goods of financial trade, markets induce us to treat people as a means rather than as an end in themselves, thereby violating the sacrosanct maxim to respect all persons at all times. The market naturally heightens our motivation to participate in practices corrupted by the self-interested prospect of profit.[42] Hungarian philosopher Karl Polanyi has argued that commodities interrupt important social relations and supplant them with surrogates absent the depth and meaning with which such goods are normally associated.[43] Along these lines, Jeffery Stout puts the corrupting nature of commodification to a sharper point:

> Like the practice of voting, the activity of buying commodities on the market tends to reduce the results of our practical reasoning to an expression of preferences. In the end, we purchase this, but not that, and we are prepared to pay this much, but no more. The money we are willing to spend to acquire a certain product, rent someone's services, or produce a certain outcome assigns a quantifiable public value to it, which can then be compared on a single, graduated scale to all other things assigned value in the same currency. . . . The worry being expressed about commodification has to do with a perceived tendency for a culture surrounding a capitalist market to be corrupted by the attitudes and forms of reasoning appropriate to monetary transactions. The worry is that the capitalist market is encroaching on practices in which our deepest concerns are expressed and cultivated. To attribute sacred value to something is to imply that its value can neither be measured exhaustively in quantitative terms, nor reduced to utility, nor subjected at someone's whim to trade-offs of the sorts that markets are designed to facilitate.[44]

A gift remains a gift, with value substantively assigned by the giver in a private context. By contrast, a purchased commodity has a public utility that is capped by the going market rate, stripping the original possessor of both its full ownership and the set of rituals and symbolic meanings attendant to that ownership. Moreover, commodification erodes important, communally shared values in deference to individual purchasing power and the often arbitrary favoring of goods that accompany individuals' choices.

This perhaps explains why commodification is often identified as a kind of idolatry, and why those who subscribe to a "sanctity of life" doctrine warn that commodification will result in human arrogance and failure to recognize what is rightly to be considered the purview of the Divine. According to many theological worldviews, we are the stewards but not owners of our bodies. Our bodies are not ours to sell, value, dispense with, or treat with anything short of the proper reverence a curator would exhibit over a precious item on loan to a world-class museum. It is no accident that the history of the field of bioethics, devoted in large part to exploring the limits of human autonomy in the era of technological advance, is populated by scholars who emerged out of the disciplines of theology and religious studies.[45] There are grounds to consider the ethics of organ donation alongside more standard issues in bioethics such as abortion, euthanasia, stem cell research, and human cloning, all of which have in common the matter of the seriousness with which created matter is treated. The literature addressing the skepticism about selling organs from the point of view of "sanctity of life" is vast, and there is no need to rehearse it here. However, it is worth noting that a permissive attitude toward the creation of a market for organ sale stands in tension with the communitarian worldview espoused by many religious traditions.[46] Assigning a monetary value to a bodily organ arguably empowers the human being in a manner inappropriate to his dominion, just as does deciding whether embryos can ever be discarded or used for purposes other than for the creation of new life.

Even if one remains theologically agnostic, the general problem of the circumstances under which individual preference should be permitted to encroach on shared communal values remains a problem for the proponent of legalizing the sale of organs. Whether or not one believes God is the creator of all life, there are consequences to assuming that it is one's absolute right with which to do what one wants with one's own kidney. This is because such a decision cannot be made in a vacuum. A woman's choice to abort her fetus, whether morally permissible or not, affects more than the woman deciding on any particular occasion. Likewise, there is an inevitable value-impact for extending the bounds of permissibility in the instance of organ procurement. Thus Stout and others worry about a capitalist market that rubs up against practices that socially reflect the manner in which our "deepest concerns" are "expressed and cultivated." Certain communal values, theological or otherwise, cannot be sustained in a society in which individual preference always assumes the highest priority.

More specifically, commodification alters the nature of gift-giving and invites other social consequences. It is worth considering the extent to which we have the right to form and become known for harboring certain identities consistent with our most cherished beliefs. What might happen to my set of values and internal motivation if I am deprived, through legislation, of putting myself in situations in which I can spontaneously or monumentally arrive to help another in need? Radin identifies this as a consequence of losing a coveted "inalienable" status otherwise assigned to certain valuable goods.[47] We lose control over our ability to designate the things over which we retain precious stewardship for noble purposes if the society in which we are embedded pulls the rug out from under us by no longer identifying these things as precious. As bioethicist James Childress argued when he vice-chaired the National Organ Task Force on Organ Procurement and Transplantation in the mid-1980s, at stake in legalizing the sale of organs is our conception of personhood and the ability to develop the impulse of dignity we may discover within ourselves.[48] If Childress is correct, then placing limits on what we have the right to do with our bodies removes other important barriers to becoming flourishing individuals that exist in our world. Again, whether or not legislation ought to be enacted to permit the sale of organs, commodification has an effect on our social relations as well as on our ability to become certain sorts of persons and flourish.

Even if we grant that capitalist incentives have a positive net effect on the procurement of organs, we still must decide whether or not we would want to live in a society that allows the practice. To consider making such a change with any kind of civic seriousness, we would have to look at a series of correlations between the effect of monetization and the prevalence of practices that cement trust between individuals in communal settings. A society in which the commodification of any good becomes fair game, whatever else it is, reflects a commitment to values that are different than the ones we have at present, and the change will affect our prospects for communal flourishing.

To reinterpret as fungible something that previously was considered deeply personal, precious, and arguably "sacred," then, impedes and might even prevent gift-giving and other related practices that are tantamount to the formation of identities compatible with some shared visions of the good. As Radin notes, while bestowing commodities gives the giver the practical latitude of flexibility, there is a danger that the gift will come to be thought of as a "bargain"—that is, an exchange wherein "something I value yields me monetizable value in return" that endorses a "picture of persons as profit-maximizers."[49] Like a powerful spice that comes to define the whole dish once introduced, there is no putting the commodified genie back in the bottle, where it might hypothetically reclaim some of its sentimental or personal value. A policy shift in deference to capitalism and individualism in this sense ironically brings about a final, communal value: the value that a thing's bottom line worth is to be indistinguishable from its price tag. This is a consequence that, among other things, leads to the distinct issue of the effect of commodification on public perception.

A true story about trade in tissue will help clarify that when we consider the commodification of organs without proper regard for the reception of a new policy, we do so at our own peril. It is presently legal in this country to profit from trade in human tissue only when that tissue is earmarked for biotechnology, medical supplies, or other commercial products and not designated for reinsertion into another human body (e.g., for a cornea or a torn anterior cruciate ligament transplant). As stories run by the *Orange County Register* and *Chicago Tribune* in the spring and summer of 2000 made embarrassingly clear, such tissue designated for commercial use is usually procured from unsuspecting families who, in giving permission for the bodies of their deceased loved ones to be used for lifesaving transplantation or for general use in anatomical research, also unwittingly sign away the rest of their body parts to industry, which hospitals and other healthcare institutions make available for a price.[50]

Take the example of skin procured from deceased donors in which approval by the donor's family is customarily obtained under fine print most likely ignored at the time the organ donor card is signed. Some of this skin is used to make Alloderm, a product initially developed to treat burn victims but which has, over time, come to be used by plastic surgeons for the purpose of removing facial wrinkles, enlarging and changing the shape of lips, and making cosmetic improvements elsewhere on the body, including the genital area.[51] Not surprisingly, when the *Register* broke the story and reported this, people were outraged.

An investigation led the US Department of Health and Human Services to refine its regulations regarding tissue trade in the United States, but the publicity consequences, despite subsequent modification to policy, were disastrous at the time the article appeared. Although the exposed abuses dealt with tissue only, campaigns calling attention to the cause of organ transplantations also suffered a setback. Public buy-in again became a tough sell as a result of what many felt was a duplicitous infringement on their personal autonomy by the commercial industry. As noted in the last chapter, during the early 1980s, around the time of the passage of NOTA, the transplantation industry successfully convinced a resistant public by framing organ transplantation as a virtuous option that opened up possibilities for creating a special bond between donor and recipient. This characterization got a sales boost when Pope John Paul II included organ donation as part of his agenda on behalf of the "culture of life" in his *Evangelium Vitae* in 1995.

The abuse of the public's trust in this and other instances of profit-taking from the sale of tissue that is precariously procured put this rationale in jeopardy. Some felt the transplantation industry had treated them like fools.[52] There is a larger point, however: that with commodification this sort of thing is bound to happen, and when it does it will undermine the grounds on which people's trust is historically earned—that is, the grounds of transparency, honesty, and fairness that govern the proposed lifesaving other-regarding gesture. Bad stories in the press also add fuel to the fire for individuals bent on perpetuating myths about the practice of organ donation for their own reasons, including the damaging myth that hospitals do not do due diligence in guaranteeing that the "dead donor rule" (organs are procured from deceased bodies only) is scrupulously followed every time.[53]

Making the sale of bodily organs legal, and the casual way in which body parts can come to be regarded as fungible or transferable like other goods, can have dreadful consequences for a society's continued acceptance of the practice of organ donation more generally because such a policy shift complicates the narrative by which initial objections to the practice are overridden in the name of the perceived noble spirit of "giving the gift of life." This is not to say that self-interest and altruism are opposed to one another. To the contrary, the current system of donation is fueled by a realization that it *does* matter to people that they can not only give but be perceived as giving, which, research shows, motivates future giving in different contexts. As the sociologist Roberta Simmons observes in her work on donor motivation, we must distinguish "venal or pathological motives from motives associated with 'subtle self-rewards,' such as the desire for one's life to matter, to improve one's self-picture, to feel happier about life and self, to relieve the distress of empathy with the victim, or to obey religious and societal norms. When these subtle self-rewards or societal pressures operate *along* with empathy, the helping act remains admirable."[54]

While a purist like the philosopher Immanuel Kant might quarrel with this plurality of motives driving a helping act, many religious and secular thinkers, including Aristotle, acknowledge that self-flourishing is completely consistent with, and in fact is the other side of the coin of, other-regard.[55] The problem with commodification is that the introduction of money comes to govern the entirety of the donor's motivation, precisely precluding the sort of healthy, complementary balance maintained between self-flourishing and other-regard.

As previously noted, often we have a perception problem because there is a real problem. It is a tenuous and often messy thing to tinker with long-standing social mores that support people seeing themselves in a positive light and aspiring to interact with others as their best selves. But, again, moving beyond perception and putting this pragmatic concern aside, there is also a strictly ethical worry that policy changes can trigger our baser instincts and, like a malignancy, come to dominate our inner motivational operating system enough that we scarcely have the chance to become our better selves. Rewards intended to appeal exclusively to self-interest, as they are in cases of commodifying especially precious goods, do corrupt. Such appeals poison the prospect of arriving at a healthy and homeostatic balance of self-interest and altruism and as motives that can both coexist and serve one another.

Credible ethical judgments should not be made in a vacuum; they should take into account the kinds of beings we actually are. Human beings are not angels. Just as we are commonly susceptible to eating foods that are bad for us, we are susceptible to taking an easy way out when that way is presented. It is natural to jump at a chance to make money quickly if the opportunity presents itself. This does not make us bad people, but it might indicate that it is bad business, ethically speaking, to craft policies that lead us to act on naturally existing but avoidable impulses to be complacent or expedient.

MOVING FROM ETHICAL TO PRAGMATIC CONSIDERATIONS

Whether or not a policy of making organs available for sale is likely to increase the pool of available organs, there may nevertheless be strong ethical reasons for rejecting this policy anyway. These ethical considerations, however, do bear on the larger question posed here—namely, what can and should be done to stem the tide of the organ shortage crisis. Ethical misgivings feed into a thesis about motivating the activity of giving for the sake of the other in which an altruistic incentive is ultimately more effective than one based primarily on self-interest. In other words, whereas ethical reflection sometimes gives us pause in following through on solutions that otherwise seem to address our thorniest problems, in the case of the organ shortage crisis, ethical and pragmatic concerns are in lockstep. This is because of who human beings fundamentally are. Capitalism, which may be an efficient, effective, and even morally sustainable system with respect to the exchange of most goods, is not so with respect to the exchange of especially precious goods.

This conclusion has much to do with how we see ourselves. Adding a price tag to any good makes an overt, public determination about what the economic and presumably final value of that good can be. In this respect commodification closes off options. It subsumes the act of gift-giving within a system of reciprocity in which "added" values, such as sentimentality, or extra considerations, such as those that proceed from a giver of limited means, are to be counted for less than they otherwise should or could be. Commodification reduces the phenomenon of exchanging goods to isolated events of rational bartering, which in essence removes the social context and fellowship that often accompanies such exchanges. Hence the sociologist and anthropologist Pierre Bourdieu identifies in the gift exchange a "taboo of making things explicit."[56] The second we start counting and recording in society who gives what and how much this or that gift is worth, we deprive ourselves and others of the ability to act with largesse and to see each other and our acts as impulses that spring from genuine concern. When we cannot benefit from momentum that is generated when acting from a purely giving spirit, we also hamper our collective ability to "pay it forward." Bourdieu intriguingly recognizes the acceptability of sometimes *misvaluing* things in systems not based on reciprocal, recorded exchange. To be sure, with the leeway that subjective valuing of things opens up, we are afforded the opportunity to create both true and fictional narratives on which we psychologically depend—and are able *not* to see each other as calculators whose ulterior motives in interacting with others is always to further our own ends. We have a psychological need, in other words, to be able to see ourselves and others as authentic givers (which is not to say that we are never authentically assuming these roles).

This set of concerns about creating a market for the sale of organs, based on ethical and pragmatic considerations, feeds into an understanding of giving and selflessness in which our sacrifices for others are to be assigned neither an objective monetary value nor bestowed anonymously. It is additionally consistent with an understanding of altruism that should not be conflated with nor opposed to self-interest; this might be identified as "self-regarding altruism."[57] There are rewards to giving quite apart from, and indeed might be prevented by, explicit monetary rewards. According proper respect to this observation will have an impact on policies that in the long run might turn out to be most effective in recruiting willing, living donors.

NOTES

1. Ethan Gutmann, *The Slaughter: Mass Killings, Organ Harvesting, and China's Secret Solution to Its Dissident Problem* (New York: Prometheus, 2014).

2. See, for example, David Petechuk, *Organ Transplantation (Health and Medical Issues Today)* (Westport, CT: Greenwood, 2006), 79.

3. Ibid. Not surprisingly, those who subscribe to the view that the commodification of bodily organs should be prohibited on the basis of sanctity of life also find practices as various as prostitution, drug abuse, suicide, abortion, euthanasia, research on embryonic stem cells, and human cloning as deeply problematic.

4. The price tag reflects the average going rate for brokers who peddle a kidney on the international black market. Many prognosticators estimate that, were kidneys to be for sale in a legalized setting, they would retain roughly the same value, assuming that the costs associated with implementing safety precautions in a regulated system would be offset by the removal of inflation characteristic of black market pricing. For more on the figure of $150,000 in the black market, see Shmuly Yanklowitz, "Give a Kidney, Get a Check," *Atlantic,* October 27, 2015, http://www.theatlantic.com /business/archive/2015/10/give-a-kidney-get-a-check/412609.

5. This assumes, as do most market economists, that insurance or Medicare would pay for the cost of transplantations and related medical costs but not the donor's additional lump-sum reward.

6. Ursula K. Le Guin, *The Ones Who Walk Away from Omelas* (Mankato, MN: Creative Education, 1993).

7. Ibid., 32.

8. This phrase, invoking a moral issue in its very title, comes from Renée C. Fox and Judith Swazey, *Spare Parts: Organ Replacement in American Society* (Oxford: Oxford University Press, 1992).

9. S. M. Rothman and D. J. Rothman, "The Hidden Cost of Organ Sale," *American Journal of Transplantation* 6, no. 7 (2006): 1527–28.

10. Kieran Healy, *Last Best Gifts: Altruism and the Market for Human Blood and Organs* (Chicago: University of Chicago Press, 2006), 70.

11. Rothman and Rothman, "Hidden Cost of Organ Sale," 1526.

12. Ibid., 1527.

13. Harvey Wasserman, "California's Deregulation Disaster," *Nation,* January 26, 2001, http://www.thenation.com/article/californias-deregulation-disaster/.

14. R. W. Evans, "Money Matters: Should Ability to Pay Ever Be a Consideration in Gaining Access to Transplantation?," in *The Ethics of Organ Transplants: The Current Debate*, ed. Arthur L. Caplan and Daniel H. Coelho (Amherst, NY: Prometheus, 1998), 232.

15. Ibid., 233.

16. Lawrence Cohen, "Where It Hurts: Indian Material for an Ethics of Organ Transplantation," *Daedalus* 128, no. 4 (Fall 1999): 135–65, mentioned by Debra Satz, *Why Some Things Should Not Be For Sale: The Moral Limits of Markets* (Oxford: Oxford University Press, 2010), 200.

17. Satz, *Why Some Things*, 200.

18. Ibid., 200–201.

19. Madhav Goyal, Ravindra L. Mehta, Lawrence J. Schneiderman, and Ashwini R. Sehgal, "Economic and Health Consequences of Selling a Kidney in India," *Journal of the American Medical Association* 288, no. 13 (2002): 1590.

20. Ibid.

21. Ibid., 1591.

22. Ibid.

23. Ibid., 1592.

24. J. Randall Boyer, "Gifts of the Heart . . . and Other Tissues: Legalizing the Sale of Human Organs and Tissues," *BYU Law Review* no. 1 (2012): 327.

25. Peter Lawler, quoted in a discussion among the President's Council on Bioethics, chaired by Edmund Pellegrino, from a transcript in a session dated June 22, 2006, "Organ Transplantation and Procurement: The Ethical Challenge." See https://bioethicsarchive.georgetown.edu/pcbe/transcripts/june06/session3.html.

26. Boyer, "Gifts of the Heart," 313.

27. Carmella M. Kuhnen and Brian Knutson, "The Neural Basis of Financial Risk Taking," *Neuron* 47 (2005): 763–70.

28. As reported by xinhuanet.com on April 6, 2012, http://news.xinhuanet.com/english/china/2012–04/06/c_131511582.htm.

29. Goyal et al., "Economic and Health Consequences," 1591.

30. Yosuke Shimazono, "The State of International Organ Trade: A Provisional Picture Based on Integration," *Bulletin of the WHO* 85, no. 12 (2007). See http://www.who.int/bulletin/volumes/85/12/06–039370/en/.

31. Boyer, "Gifts of the Heart," 328.

32. For a discussion of the set of ethical issues surrounding "high-risk" donors, particularly in the case of serious contagious diseases, see Robert M. Veatch and Lainie F. Ross, *Transplantation Ethics*, 2nd ed. (Washington, DC: Georgetown University Press, 2015), 215.

33. Boyer, "Gifts of the Heart," 328.

34. Healy, *Last Best Gifts*, 89.

35. National Academies Institute of Medicine, *HIV and the Blood Supply: An Analysis of Crisis Decision-Making* (Washington, DC: National Academy Press, 1995), 41, cited in Healy, *Last Best Gifts*, 90.

36. Before accepting the correlation between the purity of donor motive and the recipient's health consequences too easily, some qualification is in order. Despite the fact that paying for blood tends to attract individuals at risk of contaminating the blood supply, we should not be so quick to assume, with Titmuss, that contamination occurred *because* they were paid. As Kieran Healy notes, whether or not price is to be causatively associated with a contaminated blood supply depends on the prior overlap between populations that are prevalent with disease and those where blood is allowed to be sold. For example, a society in which disease is prevalent and blood is not for sale carries more risk of contamination than one in which the population is generally healthy and blood can be for sale. See Healy, *Last Best Gifts*, 91.

37. Neelam Dhingra, "In Defense of WHO's Blood Donation Policy," *Science* 342, no. 6159 (2013): 691–92.

38. Margaret Jane Radin, *Contested Commodities: The Trouble with Trade in Sex, Children, Body Parts, and Other Things* (Cambridge, MA: Harvard University Press, 1996), xi.

39. Ibid., 97.

40. Healy, *Last Best Gifts*, 4. See also Michael Sandel, *What Money Can't Buy: The Moral Limits of Markets* (New York: Farrar, Straus, and Giroux, 2013).

41. Alasdair Macintyre, *After Virtue: A Study in Moral Theology*, 2nd ed. (Notre Dame, IN: Notre Dame University Press, 1984), 185–88.

42. Immanuel Kant, *The Groundwork of the Metaphysics of Morals*, trans. H. J. Paton (New York: Harper and Row, 1964), 92.

43. The classic statement of this view, as Healy notes, is presented by the political economist Karl Polanyi, in *The Great Transformation: The Political and Economic Origins of Our Time* (Boston: Beacon, 1980). See also Healy, *Last Best Gifts*, 5.

44. Jeffrey Stout, *Blessed Are the Organized: Grassroots Democracy in America* (Princeton, NJ: Princeton University Press, 2010), 219.

45. There are literally hundreds of articles establishing the rise of bioethics as a field and discipline as a response to the rapidly growing rate of technology in the twentieth century. For one good article summarizing the early influences, including the early role theology and religion played in shaping the field, see M.L.T. Stevens, "The History of Bioethics: Its Rise and Significance," Elsevier Inc., at https://static1 .squarespace.com/static/55563925e4b08c2f72677221/t/557884ede4b09999bf 211755/1433961709057/The_20History_20of_20Bioethics-Its_20Rise_20and_20 Significance.pdf. Stevens provides a terrific bibliography as well.

46. Objections to organ transplantation, usually based on refusal to accept brain death, abound in various religious traditions and subtraditions in the West; however, the consensus among scholars is that every major religious tradition contains ample resources to support the practice. See Veatch and Ross, *Transplantation Ethics*, 17–18.

47. Radin, *Contested Commodities*, 16, 80.

48. James Childress, "Ethical Criteria for Procuring and Distributing Organs for Transplantation," in *Organ Transplantation Policy: Issues and Prospects*, ed. J. F. Blumstein and F. A. Sloan (Durham, NC: Duke University Press, 1989), 101, 110.

49. Radin, *Contested Commodities*, 93.

50. Healy, *Last Best Gifts*, 110–11.

51. Ibid., 111–12.

52. Ibid., 118.

53. An example of a sloppy but popular publication spreading myths about physicians and organ providers who "blur" the line between alive and dead is Dick Teresi, *The Undead: Organ Harvesting, the Ice-Water Test, Beating-Heart Cadavers— How Medicine Is Blurring the Line between Life and Death* (New York: Pantheon, 2012). Teresi mischaracterizes transplant surgeons as greedy vultures, and he fails to acknowledge both that standard protocols are adhered to in every major transplantation facility in the United States and that physicians caring for a dying patient

are strictly separated from procurement teams responsible for retrieving organs after death. This noted, the example of Teresi's specious claims does call attention to the ease with which myths get spread and are given an unfortunate hearing, a situation not helped by the commercial side of tissue exchange, where many of the main players are far less scrupulous than physicians and staffs at healthcare facilities involved in the transplantation of human organs.

54. Roberta G. Simmons, "Presidential Address on Altruism and Sociology," *Sociological Quarterly* 32, no. 1 (1991): 16.

55. Andrew Michael Flescher and Daniel L. Worthen, *The Altruistic Species: Scientific, Philosophical, and Religious Perspectives of Human Benevolence* (West Conshohocken, PA: Templeton, 2007), esp. 165–200.

56. Pierre Bourdieu, *Practical Reason* (Stanford, CA: Stanford University Press, 1998), 95–97. Discussed in Healy, *Last Best Gifts,* 115.

57. Rupert Jarvis, "Join the Club: A Modest Proposal to Increase Availability of Donor Organs," in *The Ethics of Organ Transplants: The Current Debate*, ed. Arthur L. Caplan and Daniel H. Coelho (Amherst, NY: Prometheus, 1998), 190.

3

Organ Donation, Financial Motivation, and Civic Duty

PAYING IT FORWARD

Despite possible logistical difficulties at the stage of implementation of a program for selling organs, regulation can go a long way toward protecting the interests of and offering some assurances to the most vulnerable and impoverished donors who enter the marketplace. Furthermore, given the advance of technology, we are no longer quite as reliant on social histories to tell us whether a transplantation should proceed as planned. A donor's suitability to be matched with a recipient is now reinforced by a slew of independent medical tests that can be relied on to assure the safety of individuals poised to undergo a nephrectomy or receive a new kidney. Finally, it seems disingenuous to have arbitrary policies that permit some valuable goods to be exchanged in a market while prohibiting other similar ones from doing the same. There are, therefore, some good arguments to be made for the compatibility of an intrinsic, altruistic motivation for sacrifice with an extrinsic financial one, and thus an argument for regarding the creation of a market for solving the organ shortage problem as an approach that can assist the current voluntary one. Even so, it is clear that none of these issues are open and shut cases. Intelligent people can and do come at these ethical questions from different directions.

Even if all of the ethical issues were addressed to our satisfaction, however, there remains the major question of whether modifying the National Organ Transplantation Act of 1984 to allow for the sale of organs would in fact increase the number of organs available. This is a question that puts the concepts of "compensation" and "motivation"—that is, the notions of economics and psychology—at front and center. The question is largely empirical. How can we measure the effect that extrinsic (in this case financial) incentives have on inducing costly, other-regarding, impactful behaviors? This inquiry is complicated by the reality that we have no actual studies measuring the effect that the legalization of selling and buying organs on the recruitment of willing donors will have, since the practice has always been illegal in the United States and is presently illegal almost everywhere else too.

There are essentially two ways of reviewing the social sciences literature to respond to this problem and infer some conclusions: we can either look at similar sorts of cases for which we do have reliable data or we can use a method known as "econometrics," an area of economics that deploys mathematical models to make predictions. Econometrics uses statistical methods and selects variables that stand in for choice-determinants. Through the assignment of coefficients that reflect the importance of these choice-determinants to an overall equation, an informed conclusion can be derived, such as the strategic effectiveness of certain proposed policy shifts.[1]

Econometrics also can be used to test the viability of economic models, such as "rational actor" theory, which posits social behavior as a function of an aggregate of individual choices.[2] According to rational actor theory, whether or not we are likely to become organ donors would depend on the effect that introducing financial incentives will have on our self-regarding preferences. In order to assess this claim responsibly, however, the inquirer must make some effort to understand the relationship between individual motivation and collective action, which in reality is considerably more complex than it is imagined by anyone who thinks motivation is in every case reducible to incentivization based on reward.[3] To get at the question of what effect money has on motivation in cases involving costly sacrifice for the sake of rendering an especially precious good, we will have to rely on the expertise and findings of social scientists who have studied examples from the real world that are similar and relevant to the case of paying for organs and those who have worked from mathematical models designed to shed further light on the topic.

One of the more interesting things to learn from the social science literature is that how an appeal is made, or, to be more precise, how it is framed, matters. Whether we are being asked to consider a policy that allows us to be paid for donating a kidney or we are being probed to see if we are okay with a nuclear waste facility being built in proximity to where we live, if we feel that in being asked that we are also being "bought," the psychological feeling that results could trigger a reaction different from the kind of response we might have had had we been asked solely on the basis of an appeal to neighborly fellowship. Furthermore, how well we know each other and, in turn, how connected we feel to one another, makes a difference. Money is less likely to sway us if we feel less taken advantage of by those in our midst.

By contrast, it is more likely to attract our attention if we feel others are out for themselves only. Race and class are among the variables that affect this determination, and in general the predictive success of civic-minded versus financial appeals is itself multifactorial. It is thus important not to assume a result at the outset, because the answer will depend on more than one variable. In other words, offering money will not always help the cause but, by the same token, under particular circumstances civic duty will not be enough to change the minds of individuals who have reason to be suspicious before they are asked to do something costly. The success of these two strategies is contingent on the environments in which they are being deployed.

It is important to understand the impact some of these variables will have on behavior, especially in instances in which solutions to social problems require one person or a group of people to help one another. A couple of anecdotes might set the stage. The first involves a minor car accident I had on Long Island's Northern State Parkway. No one was hurt, but the other driver's car was totaled, and my car had $5,700 worth of damage. I'd had a terrible day, was late for an important meeting, and was not in the best mood even before my car was rear-ended. Emerging from our vehicles after the accident to exchange insurance information, I'm sure I wasn't donning my most welcoming or gracious expression, but the nineteen-year-old college student who hit me disarmed me immediately by the way in which he seemed to be concerned only with whether or not I was physically okay. In an instant his question transformed my mind: he changed from being an adversary to just a fellow sojourner in busy traffic. We'd both have to wait nearly forty-five minutes for the police to arrive (since we were the only accident among many accidents that evening that didn't have any reported injuries). During the wait we got to know one another as people rather than as potential litigants.

The second incident, which happened the next morning, took me by surprise even more. I was rushing to get to a meeting and felt more caffeine deprived than usual. Amid my harried state of mind waiting in line at the coffee drive-thru I was made to forget everything that seemed important when the driver of the car in front of me picked up the tab for my coffee. This was an item for purchase of just over two dollars, but the impact of the good-natured gesture, coming as it did on the heels of the one the evening before, changed the rest of my week. Together the events shook me out of the short-term state of self-absorption from which I had been suffering and opened my eyes to possibilities I might have in coming hours or days to "pay it forward" myself. But what struck me as important about the shift in my state of mind, relevant to our discussion here, is something else.

In the moments before I was hit and even in my rush to get coffee and make it to a meeting, I was in what might be characterized as a "counting" mode. Perhaps because of how I'd felt I was being treated by various people during some recent interactions, I was more than keenly aware of what was being taken from me relative to what I was being given. I was defensively postured and vigilant. But these two strangers showed me by example what it means to take the leap of faith to believe that humanely interacting with others is both its own reward and an impulse that pays dividends. When the driver who rear-ended me showed me that he wasn't foremost concerned about insurance implications (a rarity in the case of any accident on Long Island), I was no longer concerned about who would pay for the damage to my car. When a stranger bought me a coffee the next morning I acquired the temperament to stay silent during the meeting I was rushing to attend, a meeting where, as it turns out, my silence was beneficial to a good outcome.

The two events led me to involve myself helpfully in the affairs of others in the coming days—in a way that made a real difference—and, more important, afforded me the blessing of influencing them as these two drivers had influenced me. No longer preoccupied with "counting" insufficient deference or respect, I was now freed up to make sure that the shared space I inhabited with others became collectively better. The examples showed me that one's individual needs are not the most important thing, which fundamentally changed my attitude about the events themselves (that is, dealing with the aftermath of an accident and getting properly caffeinated ahead of a big meeting). That twelve-hour period changed my attitude in life as well, at least for a stretch of time. So what does all this have to do with the empirical question of whether paying someone to donate an organ will drive that person to do so?

The answer has to do with the nature of money. As Amy Friedman has often remarked, "donors shouldn't bear risks without compensation."[4] While true enough, this attitude sidesteps the real question, which is: What *sort* of "compensation" is rightly to be regarded as the most powerful and effective at motivating participation? Friedman assumes that money is it, particularly in a capitalist society such as the United States, where we learn at a young age that payment is the appropriate result of working hard, rendering a service, and exhibiting other forms of merit.

There are two problems with this assumption, though. First, as evident in the examples that follow, the introduction of money to an exchange of a good tends to put people on alert rather than relaxing them or drawing the transacting parties closer to one another. Compensation in the form of money makes us preoccupied with, if not overtly defensive about, our own well-being, sometimes to the point that we become myopically protective of our assets. Second, the idea that only money can counterweigh against a cost born of a noble sacrifice underestimates the effectiveness of nonmonetary forms of compensation. The experience of giving itself, for example, is a form of compensation. When we sacrifice for others by donating an organ to someone in need, benefits abound in several ways, including the experience of increased self-worth following donation.[5] Giving and receiving are activities that foster trust and forge bonds, and, furthermore, lead to an experience of a powerful "high" for both parties.[6] It is doubtful that such an emotionally uplifting state would be available to one getting paid for one's gift, or that a recipient would be as inclined to share in the giver's joy at having performed the lifesaving gesture. In these observations, I do not deny Friedman's point about linking risk to compensation. I am, rather, questioning what constitutes legitimate, effective compensation.

Finally, even if we determine that monetary inducements do influence the recruitment of willing living donors, we must also investigate whether those inducements stand in tension with nonmonetary compensations. If so, this tension undercuts any gains in the number of individuals inclined to act from civic duty and fellowship that the introduction of money will push away. This phenomenon is described as the "crowding-out" effect, the kernel of Richard Titmuss's observation when he compared blood donation rates in the United States and the United Kingdom.[7] Titmuss accounted for the better donation rates in England and Wales by calling attention to all of the potential voluntary donors in the United States who chose not to show up for blood drives because other donors were getting paid to do the very same thing.

According to the crowding-out thesis, price incentives created for a good formerly exchanged only through gift-giving undermine the sense of responsibility one feels to give to one's neighbor and thereby lessens everyone's openness to doing those good things they might have done gratis.[8] If the crowding-out thesis is true, then it is not enough merely to point out that altruism serves as a powerful motivation for leading people to sacrifice for the sake of others. According to Titmuss, this motivation must also be understood as an either-or situation with financial incentives. A market for organ trade cannot exist *alongside* effective campaigns that enlist volunteers to do the same. It is time to look at some concrete examples in order to come to an informed judgment about what the effects are of offering financial incentives to encourage civic sacrifice. Is Titmuss's hypothesis, intended to explain the difference in blood donation rates in different regions of the world during the middle of the twentieth century, generalizable to other cases?

WOLFENSCHIESSEN, SWITZERLAND

It is a methodological challenge to speak intelligibly about the predicted success of a proposed policy that at present remains illegal. We nevertheless might learn something about how well a market for organ trade could work by examining the impact money has had in convincing the participation of individuals currently on the fence in other real-world situations. One such case, conducted by the economist Bruno Frey and colleagues, examined the difficulty of securing sufficient space to house a nuclear waste facility in Switzerland during June of 1993.[9]

Switzerland is presently tenth in the world in terms of its reliance on nuclear energy as a percentage share of domestic electricity generation, a notably high figure for such a relatively small country; it needs to find adequate space for nuclear waste disposal.[10] (The United States ranks fifteenth). Twenty years ago, when the Swiss government sought to expand its nuclear energy program, it had a problem finding a site for a waste facility large enough and far enough away from population centers to meet its expected energy needs. Weighing several factors, especially public safety, it put considerable effort into finding the appropriate location, ultimately determining that it would be best to build it into a mountain right in the center of the country, near no major population centers, closest to the small town of Wolfenschiessen.

Believing in the value of transparency, the Swiss government admirably commissioned a representative to contact the approximately two thousand people (640 families) who lived in Wolfenschiessen to see if they were okay with the proposal. After being told about the minimal health dangers and long-term economic consequences of the proposed siting, the representative convened a large town hall–style meeting to gauge the feelings of the townspeople. In order to build a repository, the developer, the federal parliament, and those who attended the town hall all had to agree to the project. As Frey reports, "A bare majority (50.8 percent) of citizens living in the host community indicated they would support this siting decision."[11]

The first thing to notice about this figure is how high it is: 50.8 percent reflects stronger support than what most people would likely guess. Given the health and economic risks, one might have expected more resistance to the idea. Indeed, Wolfenschiessen's citizens were not shy about mentioning their specific concerns: almost 40 percent of the respondents thought the risk of an unplanned calamitous event at the repository resulting in groundwater contamination was significant, and a third (34 percent) believed that at least some residents would die as a result of this contamination. About 80 percent reportedly expressed concerns that a critical mass of town residents would suffer some sort of long-term health damage.[12] Still, a majority ultimately supported the siting proposal. It is not an overwhelming mandate, but it is impressive. Civic duty, or at least the assumption of civic responsibility on the part of those who were asked, won out over tangible and immediate self-interests.

What is perhaps even more striking about the response of the citizens, however, is what occurred when Frey and his colleagues decided to test what might be done to increase overall buy-in to the government's proposal on behalf of the Swiss people. The economists asked the townsfolk if they might accept the siting of the nuclear waste repository should the Swiss parliament decide to compensate the residents of the host community. They furthermore tried to approximate what this amount would be through a kind of calibration:

> The amount offered varied from $2,175 per individual and year (N = 117) to $4,350 (N = 102) and $6,525 (N = 86). While 50.8 percent of the respondents agreed to accept the nuclear waste repository without compensation, *the level of acceptance dropped to 24.6 percent* when compensation was offered. About one-quarter of the respondents seem to reject the facility simply because of financial compensation. The amount of compensation had no significant effect on the level of acceptance. Everyone who rejected the first compensation was then made a better offer, thereby raising the amount of compensation from $2,175 to $3,263, from $4,350 to $6,526, from $6,525 to $8,700. Despite this marked increase, only a single respondent who declined the first compensation was now prepared to accept the higher offer.[13]

There are a number of remarkable things to point out about this result. First, when Frey and his colleagues followed up with the residents of Wolfenschiessen about whether offering money might additionally incline them to become more receptive to the government's request, their positive response rate not only went down rather than up, it went down by more than half. Second, it was the introduction of money itself, and not the amount, that accounted for the change in citizens' attitudes. Only one person out of everyone surveyed felt the increase made a difference, a finding all the more significant given that the money offered was substantial and roughly comparable to the median household income per month for those surveyed ($4,565).[14] Finally, these results were not anomalous. They were not a function of, for example, some idiosyncratic feature of the town of Wolfenschiessen.

Surprised by the degree to which the introduction of financial incentives turned out to weaken from the motive for civic engagement, Frey and his colleagues decided to replicate similar versions of their survey in six communities in northeastern Switzerland. The crowding-out effect they observed in Wolfenschiessen was confirmed through the course of 206 interviews in which the sampling procedure and methodology were identical to the previous one conducted at the actual proposed site.[15] In the second iteration, a smaller percentage, 41 percent, initially stated they would vote in favor of the siting proposal, but, again, this figure dropped to 27.4 percent when money was introduced as an added incentive.[16]

These findings are not isolated to Switzerland either. As Frey notes, 498 individuals interviewed in connection with a proposed nuclear waste facility in Nevada yielded the same result, as did the results from interviews of individuals in other real and hypothetical cases.[17]

As the researchers note, more than one explanation exists for the crowding-out effect that is apparently at work in these "not in my backyard" kinds of scenarios. It is possible that the respondents were being strategic in their responses, noticing, when it occurred to them, that they potentially stood to make money and that it behooved them to start bargaining and hold out for the highest price. This was not determined to be a likely explanation, however, given how little an increase in the reward altered the results in repeated surveys.

Another explanation for the inverse relationship between financial incentives and buy-in was that the subsequent offer of money to induce more participation revealed a suspicion that the government's initial characterization of the situation was more dangerous than the government initially let on.

Frey and his colleagues, however, found this explanation wanting by testing it in a subsequent survey in which only 6.3 percent of respondents thought compensation signaled extra risk. The researchers also considered less obvious explanations for the negative impact of the introduction of financial incentives. For example, they entertained the notion that the subject of nuclear waste facilities in general makes respondents overly emotional and irrational, thus precluding their ability to trust responses at all. Again, however, follow-up surveying revealed this explanation to be inadequate.[18]

After scrutinizing and rejecting competing explanations, Frey and colleagues concluded that the phenomenon of crowding-out that Titmuss identified is the most rational and plausible reason for the erosion of civic impulses under conditions in which altruistic motivation is perceived to be the driving force of sacrifices made for the sake of a public good.[19] In a revisitation of their survey, however, they acknowledged a caveat: in a town hall vote conducted one year later, the citizens of Wolfenschiessen voted with a three-fifths majority in favor of the siting of the repository after a Swiss developer raised the compensation to the community to over $3 million per year for the next forty years, amounting to 120 percent of the community's annual tax revenue.[20]

Frey and colleagues explain this outcome as a "substitution of moral principles." The new and generous sum of money, presented as an influx of collective resources to the whole town, provided an alternative to the impression that individuals could be bought off. The idea of investing in schools, fire stations, and other shared services struck people differently than individuals receiving an allotment of money to do with what they liked.[21] Despite the fact that the developer essentially did what the economists had probed the effect of in their surveys—increase the amount of compensation—this time the people of Wolfenschiessen went for it. The difference is that the increase was not presented as an individual enticement but as a reinvestment in communal projects and goals, thereby preserving the initial civic impulse under which the offer was first considered.

HOW BUYING A GOOD CHANGES A GOOD

The Wolfenschiessen outcome is consistent with the observation that it matters to individuals how others see them and how they are able to see themselves. When we sense that others feel we can be bought, or see ourselves as being able to be bought, we acquire independent self-interested reasons for rejecting seemingly attractive outcomes that entail a personal boon or a maximization of profit. If the pitch is altered, however, we may become more receptive. Thus, as Frey and his colleagues note:

> As long as the bribe effect dominates individual expressions, verbal opposi-
> tions against noxious facilities is to be expected. In this situation, many de-
> velopers break off the negotiations hoping to find another host community
> more willing to take the project. However, compensation packages meeting
> the needs of the residents living in the prospective host community would
> show their effect only if sufficient time were allowed. Developers are able
> to minimize the *perceived* moral cost of accepting compensation by clearly
> distinguishing these financial incentives from bribes. . . . Despite loss of
> efficiency, in-kind compensation benefitting the community as a whole
> weakens the bribe effect as it evokes the notion that votes, to a lesser extent,
> are bought. (italics added)[22]

Rational economic thinking can be made to be compatible with moral principles. Acting from a virtuous impulse matters to us and makes coherent our
understanding of human fulfillment and how we relate to others. Different
kinds of incentives are therefore not always, but can be, additive. As these
surveys demonstrate, in order to preserve and benefit from the participation
of those who are intrinsically motivated to do good acts, extrinsic motivation
has to be redescribed, and arguably importantly altered, to emphasize this
intrinsic component.

The example of finding a suitable host site for a nuclear waste facility is also
instructive insofar as it gives insight into the sorts of things that are eligible
to be bought. Reflecting on these sorts of cases and similar ones, Michael
Sandel makes a distinction between the things that we perhaps shouldn't buy
but which come with a price tag and those things we can't buy without rendering the good in question incoherent. Sandel does this in order to raise the
question about the degree to which these two kinds of things are ultimately
different from one another.[23]

To begin with the latter, Sandel considers certain obvious examples: friendship (which requires genuine fellowship and closeness); education (which involves actual learning and not the mere reported evaluation of accomplished
work); and prestigious academic, professional, and sporting awards (which
are public recognitions of rare genius or athletic performance). In all of these
cases, when money buys the good it also dissolves it, since money can't buy

those aspects of the good that are earned and which gives them value. Sandel raises the interesting example of services that provide wedding toasts or funeral eulogies for purchase, rendered by the orator as if he or she had been the one to come up with the inspiration for the moving words. Any revelation that the "sentimental masterpiece" was bought changes exactly the impact it was intended to make, which is why a key feature of the purchased product is the concealment of its construction.[24]

These kinds of examples are clear enough: if the good is bought, it ceases to be. Friendship, educational or athletic milestones, and expressed sentiments of a personal nature delivered for a delicate occasion are all things that are "earned" based on things internal to the achievement itself, even if we are able to fool onlookers by purchasing the appearance of having achieved them legitimately. Commodification in these instances isn't simply discouraged; commodification is impossible to do without corrupting the purchased item itself. The good would be revealed to be worthless were the truth of its acquisition to become transparent.

Slightly but importantly different than this category of goods are those items that perhaps *shouldn't* be bought but whose acquisition, when purchased, doesn't technically render them incoherent. Sandel raises as examples purchased kidneys or babies put up for adoption. The question is whether the same contaminating influence of money is in effect similar to the cases of bought friendships or grades. Do not kidneys save lives whether they are purchased or not? Do not children represent worthy objects of parental love and affection regardless of how the relation between mother and child came to be established? Maybe such goods *shouldn't* ever be bought and sold, but they coherently can be, and when they are they fulfill the function they were intended to fill as though they had been acquired without any financial component.

However, Sandel goes on to argue, the matter is not so clear. As with the good of a society's blood banks, organs procured for reinsertion into another body or children available to be put up for adoption by a loving family are already regarded in our society as symbolic of the public character of the community in which, as goods *qua* goods, they are cherished and acknowledged. The distinction between "can't" and "shouldn't" is therefore not so clear. In the case of the good of citizens of a town stepping up to collectively sacrifice for their host nation, the donor of an organ or adopter of a baby retains the privilege of being able to shoulder a civic burden and thereby engage in the fulfilling activity of acting virtuously. If a child is sold or bought the way a pet is, there is a lingering sense that those who have come together to facili-tate this child's future well-being disappointingly chose not to do so without profiting as well. The activity of purchasing the good thereby becomes cor-rupting, for it is now an activity that strips from the good its intangible aspect of being able to showcase displays of virtue which, when witnessed in society, also strengthen that society.

This corrupting sense of paying for an especially precious good, further-more, can also be detected. Legalizing a market for adoption or the sale of organs entails transparency. If those who rendered a good under a presump-tion that they could not get paid for doing so detect, with the addition of a price tag, that that good has been stripped of its symbolic and inspirational significance, they will look for another means of being able to imbue their society with virtuous expressions. People are more complicated than those who subscribe to reductive theories about human nature imagine them to be. We are in general not psychologically hardwired to think, feel, or act as rule-following do-gooders, ceaselessly governed by a sole directive of further-ing the overall good. Human fulfillment also involves being able to form an identity, somewhat naturally, as one who participates in the process of human betterment, a process that the introduction of money inherently undercuts. *This* is how paying for babies or kidneys is corrupting.

It is thus morally and economically rational to reject attempts to convert especially precious goods into fungible items whose fair value in cash is to be determined. Aside from their tangible function, such goods also symbol-ize important social opportunities for virtue. Their conversion into fungible items of use not only shouldn't but can't take place without narrowing what the good fully represents. Making a precious good for sale, Sandel, Frey, and others suggest, changes that good from what it once was (by corrupting it) *and*, because such a change is perceived, affects the collective motivation to render the good. Specifically, financial incentives crowd out public spirit. To support this observation, Sandel discusses two case studies somewhat less mo-mentous than the siting of a nuclear waste facility: teenagers who collect char-ity and day care facilities that serve as a communal solution to the childcare needs of working families.

In the first example, economists did an experiment to see if Israeli high school students who annually go door to door on "donation day" to raise charity for worthy domestic causes would be additionally motivated when financially incentivized to bring in pledged sums of money.[25] The researchers divided the students into three groups: one receiving the usual motivational speech about the importance of the causes for which they were raising money, and the other two being offered 1 percent and 10 percent, respectively, of the money they raised (not out of their own efforts but from a separate source).[26] Consistent with an expectation we would have after examining the nuclear waste facilities siting example, the unpaid collectors raised the most money, followed by the students who were offered the higher of the two commissions. Those who were given 10 percent did significantly better than those given 1 percent of the money they raised, leading us to wonder whether if paying them even more than 10 percent would have catapulted them into the most successful group of the three. This result garnered enough attention for the researchers to title their paper "Pay Enough or Don't Pay at All."[27] The title tantalizingly suggests that while it may well be that money corrupts, or least converts, a precious good, that corruption might be worth the cost in terms of what new participation unprecedented financial enticements might spawn.[28]

Before moving to the second study, it might be helpful to reflect on a difference between the conclusions to be drawn from the examples of townsfolk considering whether to host a nuclear waste facility and teenager charity collectors. Increases in financial incentive basically made no difference in the first case but made a big difference in the second. Why is this so? The answer likely pertains to the difference between the goods in question.

The first good, which entailed both a significant cost to the givers but a benefit to the country as a whole, was resistant to being "corrupted" in the fashion Sandel has described; the second good, with the stakes relatively lower, was inherently more convertible, so much so that it could be seen by its renderer as the sort of thing (i.e., a job) for which one normally gets paid. Thus there are two thresholds in play: how precious the good in question is deemed to be, and the amount of money it takes to convert a slightly less precious good into a financial transaction. Even in the case of the lower stakes example, however, the good of collecting charity was still resistant to being incentivized by explicit promises of pay-offs, which suggests that the teens took seriously the intrinsic value of the service they were rendering. Let's look at the second case, which deals more explicitly with how the introduction of money threatens to change a good that can suddenly be bought.

Sandel led the same group of economists in a review of Israeli day care centers in which parents were increasingly tardy in picking up their children. They discovered that the introduction of fines, intended to disincentivize lateness, only exacerbated the problem. When parents discovered they were being charged extra, they began to make the most of the new service for which they were now paying, pushing to the limit the time at which they arrived to pick up their children.[29] But in this case there was a new wrinkle not yet observed in the experiments discussed so far: when the fine was removed twelve weeks later, the adults' arrival times did not improve. Apparently the introduction of money had *permanently* altered the nature of the (unstated) assumptions governing the norms and expectations of day care centers. This is significant. What presumably started out as a social good—a service funded by publicly retrieved resources for the benefit of the whole community—had changed into a good that its users now saw as a way of attending to their individual needs. Such a consequence has some of the ethical implications already discussed, but it also has fiscal ones. As Sandel notes:

> From an economic point of view, social norms such as civic virtue and public spiritedness are great bargains. They motivate socially useful behavior that would otherwise cost a lot to buy. If you had to rely on financial incentives to get communities to accept nuclear waste, you'd have to pay a lot more than if you could rely instead on the residents' sense of civic obligation. If you had to hire schoolchildren to collect charitable donations, you'd have to pay more than a 10 percent commission to get the same result that public spirit produces for free.[30]

We do more, and do more efficiently, when our better angels are activated by a (financially) cost-neutral investment in causes that are in all of our interests to promote. One of the reasons crowding out rings true as an explanation for why it is hard for altruistic and financial motives to coexist in promoting the same good is that the introduction of money supports what might be characterized as a negative impulse to look out for number one, which neutralizes the prior positive impulse of being "all in it together."

Libertarians' protests notwithstanding, markets remove what Sandel refers to as the "bargain" of coordinated behavior. They do this by disrupting the habitual nature of how in practice we come together to conserve and then promote civic virtue. As Sandel notes through reference to Aristotle and Rousseau, the transmission of virtue is a shared activity that is encouraged by participating in publicly celebrated activities, the performance of which, in turn, further spurs similar sorts of activities.[31] By its very nature the introduction of money isolates the particular good to be traded from other in-kind goods. While this may not be such a terrible thing with regard to goods that would normally accommodate commodification anyway, it does become a problem in the case of especially precious goods because in those cases the grounds for the initial buy-in on the part of the community as a whole, where sacrifice is often shared, become shaky.

Note that this economic argument is related to, but separate from, the ethical argument about why we should resist putting a price tag on some goods even if doing so were to be shown to be efficient and effective in acquiring them. Here the argument, pragmatic in nature, is that adding the price tag doesn't work for reasons that are rational, even if they don't comport with the prudentially calculating mind of a "rational actor." These examples tell us something about how successful we'd likely be in closing the organ shortage gap if we were to legalize the selling and buying of organs. *If* we perceive the activity of becoming an organ donor as something that has an individual but also important collective value, then exclusively reducing the good of a bodily organ to its individualized purpose will get in the way of overall donation as much as it will promote it.

There may be further consequences to the conversion of such a good. Studies show that public displays of civic engagement dovetail with the general level of trust present in a social setting.[32] Conversely, political and economic systems in which trust is prevented from spreading leads to the presence of freeloaders and, consequently, more distrust among the citizenry. To study this relationship, Bruno Frey measured the effect attitudes about trust among the Swiss citizenry had on displays of civic virtue by doing an econometric analysis of tax-paying behavior, looking specifically at the effect of tax morale.[33]

Trying to understand the phenomenon of freeloading, Frey assigned importance to variables in equations designed to test what conditions were optimal for inducing people to pay their taxes legally and honestly and, conversely, what conditions induced people to game the system. Variables included the percentage of income not declared, the probability of detection, the penalty for being caught, the mean marginal tax rate, and legal income deduction possibilities. By isolating these variables in hypothetical scenarios based on real data that was assembled by Swiss tax authorities, Frey established a relationship between the perception that the Swiss system of taxation was fair and the percentage of citizens correctly paying their taxes.[34]

Frey's work shows that a sense of fairness and public spirit "crowds in" participants inclined to do their own part virtuously and honestly. This crowding in depends on a cooperation that is neither forced by bureaucratization nor undermined by the sort of opportunism that surfaces when citizens are isolated from one another. The less shared goods come to assume a collective character, the more knaves and opportunists will come out of the woodwork and breed a self-perpetuating culture of distrust. Furthermore, the monetizing of a good might corrupt a particular good *and* the culture in which that good is procured. At the same time, too much regulation might squelch the human spirit that leads to public support in favor of supporting that same good. In crafting a response to both of these pressures, Frey recommends a "balanced constitution" that on the one hand is

> strict enough to effectively deter exploitative behavior, not least because it undermines civic virtue if it becomes widespread. At the same time, care must be taken to design a system of laws fundamentally trusting [of] citizens and politicians. Public laws designed for the worst possible behavior . . . run the risk of destroying the positive attitude of citizens and politicians towards their constitution which is necessary to maintain in efficiency, and is vital for its long run survival.[35]

There is no substitute, in terms of productivity, for the kind of groundswell of support for a project that a critical mass of a community needs no convincing to support. This explains why, following terrible disasters such as tornadoes and mass killings, to which most in the community can immediately and sympathetically relate, individuals tend to unite and pool their collective resources to respond to those thrust into need. The "constitutional" rules of law and government we might construct to encourage collective action should create a proper nurturing ground within which trust can sprout and develop, minimizing the likelihood that a society will experience an increase in knavery and freeloading.

This leads to an important but often neglected point about public attitudes toward providing incentives for organ donation: public resistance to legislation that supports the legalization of buying and selling organs, it turns out, is *less* strong in the case of vulnerable minority groups, particularly low-income groups.[36] The less money and standing one has, the more favorable one is likely to be to the idea of receiving reimbursement for donating one's organ(s). This is especially so in capitalistic economies, such as the United States, where disparity is more pronounced than elsewhere. Why? One way of explaining the anomaly among vulnerable or resource-poor populations is that those populations are less likely to feel supported by the larger community in general.

They may see themselves as lacking the luxury to cultivate the kind of largesse and buy-in that we have just been touting as the mark of a thriving society.

Tellingly, skepticism among vulnerable groups toward our voluntary system of procuring organ donors is also consistent with their attitudes toward other major aspects of our healthcare system.[37] For a number of reasons, including socioeconomic status and prevalence of disease within certain populations, there is a feeling among some disadvantaged groups that they are already the ones least likely to benefit from what our healthcare system has to offer.[38] This, in turn, arguably breeds a sense of distrust over many aspects of our way of providing medical resources to those most in need of them and lends support to a historical memory informed by a series of abuses over the last century that these populations have suffered at the hands of other powerful elites.[39]

Constraints of time and space prevent our delving too deeply into the question of how ethnicity, income, and race impacts attitudes about the formation of healthcare policy, but it is significant for purposes of the current discussion to call attention to what seems to be lacking in these vulnerable populations—namely, the feelings of trust and fellowship that optimize recruitment of donors in better-supported communities. Distrust, not ideal for its own reasons, is also economically disadvantageous in terms of furthering the utilitarian goals under consideration. The time and financial burdens alone with which vulnerable populations have to cope on a daily basis just to negotiate the map of our complex medical system are considerable. As Jagbir Gill and his colleagues explain, these burdens make the costs of living donation seem more immediate:

> Individuals lose the equivalent of 1 month's salary to donate a kidney, including time away from work to complete the pretransplant evaluation, hospitalization, and postsurgical convalescence. In addition to lost income, there are significant out-of-pocket expenses, including travel, lodging, and childcare, that are borne by kidney donors. Therefore, low-income potential donors may simply not be able to afford the costs of kidney donation.[40]

And the long-term costs of becoming a living kidney donor pack a greater punch with regard to these populations:

> Household income is an important socioeconomic determinant of health, with several studies outlining inferior health outcomes in lower-income

groups, including a higher risk of diabetes, coronary artery disease, obesity, psychiatric illness, and, importantly, ESRD. Furthermore, high-risk behaviors, such as tobacco and substance abuse, are more common in lower-income populations and social support networks may be poorer in these groups.[41]

It is not widely known that this demonstrable link exists between household income and health outcomes. Yet buy-in of the sort that leads to the most optimal economic outcomes hinges on a widely disseminated and transparent assumption that a society is "all in it together," so to speak. If some populations feel generally exploited within their host societies, they will be likely to retreat as a group into a more defensive posture.

There are, therefore, limitations to the economic strategy of rejecting a market approach, based on concerns about crowding out. For the strategy to work, a society largely has to be working together. A small and largely homogenous town in central Switzerland is a far cry from a contemporary urban American population characterized by diverse ethnic and income traits. That said, the same observation might be made in service of an optimistic outcome: if we systematically attend to the root causes that lead to income disparity and vulnerability among minority groups, then we might do better addressing these problems of social inequity, not piecemeal, as Veatch proposes through the narrow fix of raising the standards of the poor by giving them money for their organs, but through broad institutional reforms consistent with the tenets of social justice. If we show vulnerable populations that we care about them for real, we will earn larger societal buy-in and, in turn, a broader and more natural appeal to everyone's civic sensibilities.

The take-away message from looking at low-income and minority populations is one that complicates the conclusion to which we seem to be coming. Indeed, a policy of relying on goodwill rather than offering a monetary reward for one's kidney will in general be more successful if the society in which it is being deployed is one where trust is abundant, and where in general individuals are not wary of being mistreated, exploited, or subject to a system that leaves them feeling helpless, either with regard to experiencing poor health outcomes or in other areas where they are at risk. The introduction of financial incentives may lead to a phenomenon of crowding out, regardless, but additionally enacting policies intended to produce conditions of social justice can further help to maximize civic buy-in.

THE DIFFERENCE BETWEEN LUMP-SUM INCENTIVES AND
COMPENSATORY MEASURES

We have gone some distance in being able to make a plausible prediction about what the likely effect would be, in terms of the pragmatic goal of recruiting willing, living donors, of trying to increase participation by legalizing the sale of organs. Scrutiny of real-world scenarios involving the promotion of goods that entail significant cost to the giver (through the creation of elaborate surveys and econometric analyses) seem to suggest two things: (1) that a better outcome is more likely if we engender a robust public spirit rather than implement financial incentives; and (2) these two approaches stand in some tension with one another. However, until now we have been assuming that financial incentives take the form of large lump-sum payments. But a large one-time payment is not necessarily the same as compensatory measures designed to help alleviate the financial costs and health risks donors take on when making their sacrifice.

Compensatory measures do not, it turns out, deter intrinsic motivation and public spirit in the same manner as financial incentives do. Such payments are regarded in a categorically different light. They are not intended as inducements in themselves but rather as a means of making up for harms faced. They are designed only to make the donor's altruistic action as undisruptive as possible, in order to prevent deterrence but not entice. Correspondingly, compensatory payments do not feel like a bribe, are not subject to the "corrupting" market effect of concern to Sandel and others, and consequently do not inspire any level of general distrust that feeds into the crowding-out effect. More will be said about the ways these compensatory measures represent constructive solutions to our existing organ shortage problem. For now, it is important to describe what these measures are in order to distinguish them qualitatively from the sorts of raw financial incentives we have been discussing.

Practical solutions have recently been proposed to compensate donors for the costs they bear in making their gifts, most of which, like lump-sum payments, have financial implications. However, as the legal status of many of these compensatory measures is somewhat murky, it is unclear whether they are consistent with the spirit of the prohibition against exchanging organs for "valuable consideration" as specified in the National Organ Transplantation Act of 1984. Unlike large financial payments, however, they are not explicitly ruled out. These include providing fully comprehensive health insurance for a meaningful amount of time or for life; providing disability and life insurance for living donors (and funeral expenses to be given to the families of deceased donors); providing short- and long-term follow-up care, including access to premium health care should any complications arise from the transplant; providing modest pension contributions, tax credits, and charitable contributions in a donor's name; and additional measures intended to address the day-to-day difficulties experienced by lower-income donors.

Each of these measures was endorsed by prominent bioethicists and physicians in a letter written to then-President Barack Obama, Secretary of Health and Human Services Sylvia Mathews Burwell, Attorney General Eric Holder, and leaders of Congress.[42] Noting that our current efforts to recruit living donors are inadequate, especially in light of the growing number of individuals suffering from end-stage renal disease, the hope is that such measures will address the concerns over hardships endured with donation, particularly in vulnerable communities. It is hoped it will do so without also negatively affecting participation rates among those who are motivated by an inner sense of civic responsibility and who might be turned off by the introduction of financial incentives. Would these proposed measures be more effective than lump-sum payments at recruiting participation?

Some evidence suggests yes. In the most comprehensive literature review to date, which looked at all opinion polls conducted between 2002 and 2012 on the subject of public attitude toward financially compensating donors, Klaus Hoeyer, Silke Schicktanz, and Ida Deleuran find that while there is a consensus of weak support for living donors receiving cash and recipients supplying cash, the idea of medical expenses being covered for the living donor received strong support.[43] Looking at responses from twenty-three key studies, the researchers also determined that financial incentives, broadly stated, are more positively valued in instances when they take a nonmarket form—that is, when the exchange is "in kind" (e.g., health related); when they are provided by a third party (e.g., the government); and when they are presented as reciprocal compensation rather than as payment for services received.[44]

This conclusion is consistent with Frey's economic analyses of what factors figure into citizens weighing whether to bear a cost for the sake of the larger society. In those studies, researchers emphasize a difference between forms of payment that appear as a bribe, on the one hand, and those that appear as an offer of social good, on the other. Only the latter can legitimately be described as adequate compensation for a harm collectively endured. Hoeyer and colleagues sought to understand why the respondents of the various surveys had such across-the-board agreement on the difference between the two sorts of financial incentives, favoring one but not the other. To this end, they turned to qualitative studies to assess informants' opinions about their own bodies, their subjective views on the nature of the kind of relationships that are produced between donors and recipients in living donation scenarios, and what values they thought were in play.

As the authors describe, a picture emerges of the donor-recipient relationship being "an enduring reciprocal relationship" not easily abrogated once begun.[45] Such a relationship has properties that make it immune to being altered, even with the introduction of money. Presumably there is something qualitatively intimate about giving a body part to another, such that a payment before or after the fact cannot easily erase the memory or dilute the significance of the gift. What is more, neither donors nor recipients tend to want a modification to this relationship once it is established. Giving or receiving an organ represents one of the most momentous occasions of their lives. In contrast to what participants of anonymous exchanges report after the fact (e.g., adhering in sperm banks), recipients and donors of organs tend to remain, and want to remain, connected to one another post-transplantation.

Hence, normative values such as fairness and mutual acknowledgment figure more prominently into an understanding of living donor motivation than do direct financial incentives. As the researchers report:

The most obvious finding reflecting common modes of reasoning suggests a need to consider a conceptual shift from financial *incentives* to other perceptions of financial *means*. . . . Overall, when surveys invite members of the general public to assess procurement models, they rate direct payment and similar [financial] incentives lower than so-called altruistic donation models of the removal of disincentives. However, the surveys also indicate an acceptance of some uses of financial means in organ procurement. The reasoning found in the qualitative studies indicates that the remuneration can be seen as an expression of fairness rather than as an incentive. If people perceive the offer as fair, they are more likely to accept it. This is the case when donors get medical expenses covered instead of incurring costs as a result of their donation. While in many industrialized countries, direct medical expenses are covered by health insurance or national health care, there are still cases of under-coverage. It appears that when people opt for remuneration, the communicative effects of the exchange are valued higher than the material effects.[46]

While the public perceives direct financial incentives not to be consistent with the ideal donor-recipient relationship, indirect forms of compensation that address donor financial or medical hardship and reflect the value of fairness do not disrupt this relationship. To quite the contrary: indirect compensation is consistent with both the donor-recipient relationship and the "altruistic donation" models that seem to most effectively fuel it. Gratitude and other expressions of appreciation, personal or public, also appear to be important. The takeaway from this comprehensive review of public opinion is that while the voluntary system of living donation currently in place seems to be the most effective in terms of engendering support, this system is consistent with, and would probably even be enhanced by, additional compensatory actions intended to affirm the relationship that is established in the donor act.

These findings are also consistent with anecdotal accounts of living donors interviewed post-nephrectomy who report it was their privilege to have rendered a gift to one in need. They regard the humanizing experience entailed in their gift-giving as nonnegotiable. However, that experience is typically characterized as a two-way street: it is important to both living donors and recipients that no one be exploited in the giving process.

Lauren Muskauski, a living donor I met and interviewed, told me that while she never would have accepted significant payment for the kidney she donated as part of a paired exchange, she would accept a modest amount, perhaps a few thousand dollars, to compensate her for the financial burdens she had to incur in the donation process.[47] Moreover, she said that she would be upset if now, after she had become a donor, a new law were passed allowing donors to be directly compensated by their recipients. Despite this, she remains close to the person for whose sake she donated, and though she was never motivated to donate for money (nor would she have been), fairness, including evaluations along monetary lines, still matters to her. This particular set of concerns is consistent with a picture of the self that flourishes in the context of a community but does not dissolve amid that community. Lauren never characterized herself as a self-abrogating saint, nor as someone who wished to be denied the acknowledgment that came with her sacrifice. But she did not donate her kidney for the money either. She did it out of respect, a sense of obligation, and the love she felt for someone she cared about who was in need.

CIVIC DUTY

It is thus important that our sense of connection be preserved in the donation process, but not at the expense of forgoing fairness and due recognition on the part of heroes whose sacrifices extend and enhance the lives of those in need. This point is not completely lost on lawmakers. The National Organ Donor Leave Act of 1999 does specify provisions for allowing leave time for federal employees who are living donors, and some states have implemented laws that provide paid medical leave and tax deductions for living donors in an effort to treat donors fairly and to recruit additional ones.[48] Clearly, more along these lines needs to be considered. And whatever is done must strengthen the underlying motivation at play when individuals consider enduring a hardship for the sake of others, in the context of rendering a precious social good. That motivation remains, simply, the intrinsic urge to step up and help someone who is in significant need. This brings us to the primary alternative to the financial incentives that motivates living donor participation: civic duty.

While our current system of voluntary donation of course leaves open the door for civic engagement, the fact that it is the only legal option by which living donation is allowed does not mean that we have a donation culture of robust civic engagement. In many instances individuals who voluntarily donate for someone else do so for personal reasons that pertain to an existing relationship between the donor and the recipient. These donation scenarios often occur in individualized settings, where a recipient is lucky enough to have a specific person, usually a family member, who is willing to step up to the plate on his or her behalf. Whether we might be able to widen this circle of concern by spurring civic engagement through educational and other efforts is, to a large degree, untested.

Lest the term "civic duty" be misconstrued as imposing some binding moral obligation to put ourselves in harm's way, we should be clear that it is not an obligation that strikes us as an external sanction from the outside. Rather, civic duty properly construed is an organic, self-reinforcing communal norm that is strengthened the more it is practiced. Civic duty thus pertains to a recipient-generated inducement to care for those whose plights we know, as opposed to a moral requirement to "be a good person." When we are able to see ourselves as members of a connected society and learn more about what it means to be suffering, a sense of "ought" will begin to emanate from within that then induces us to act. It is *this* impetus to act—the action sprung from a deepening connection with the one in need—that is being proposed as a rival to the financial incentives that some believe will help with living donor recruitment.

The hypothesis on the table is that our current voluntary system for recruiting living donors, aided by a deepening sense of civic duty that is not imposed or enforced by the government or any other outside entity, can do better than any market for organ trade. According to this hypothesis, people will be most motivated to assume risk for the sake of others not because they are told to do so by a moral or religious tradition or because they stand to get paid a great deal. Rather, they will do it because they have of their own accord decided to become involved in the well-being of others. What society has so far not done a good job of doing is raising social awareness about what it means to be an organ donor and how being a donor stands to affect many different lives.

Raising social awareness means educating the public better. Many assume direct financial incentives will be what is needed in order to overcome hurdles to recruitment because of the significant costs associated with, for example, donating a kidney. Such assumptions, however, do not pay enough attention to the benefits also associated with becoming a living donor or to the way people are inspired to put the interests of others ahead of their own once they get to know them personally. While we do not have an enormous amount of research contrasting the efficacy of the competing motivations of financial incentives versus civic duty, over the last twenty years extensive research has attempted to describe and explain living donors' transplantation experiences from their own perspectives. There is ample evidence that not only do donors not regret their decisions to donate, even after weighing the costs and benefits, but they also experience an increase in self-worth, better relationships with others (including their recipients), and a happier sense of being alive.[49]

Despite these findings, however, little has been done to broadcast these advantages (in contrast to donating blood, about which there is much more awareness). In response to this absence of publicity, Amy Waterman and James Rodrigue created a list of recommendations intended both to raise public awareness about living donation and to improve the quality of education in organized media campaigns that address, head-on, both harmful popular myths about organ donation and the unheralded important benefits.[50] These include things as basic as knowing where dialysis centers are located in order to have the ability to meet a patient in need of a kidney; promoting the economic and health benefits of transplantation over dialysis; providing patient and living donor access to statewide donor exchange and donation programs; honing in on what specific barriers exist for participation among minorities and underprivileged populations; and, not least, making the intangible benefits to donors who give the gift of life widely known—for example, in celebration ceremonies praising their heroic actions.[51] Currently these sorts of campaigns occur only sporadically and not as methodically or regularly as they do in blood drives and other awareness events for comparable causes. Were such an educational program not so underdeveloped, we would have more resources available to us for recruiting willing living donors.

This noted, civic duty carries with it its own set of presumptions. Just as markets can change social norms, so too can the strengthening of norms reduce our temptation to rely on markets alone. In terms of the campaign to recruit living organ donors, the social norms that matter involve community building, fostering solidarity, and bridging the differences that exist between disparate members of that community. While the term "duty" implies a legal or moral ought of some sort, the qualifier "civic" adds a sense of the larger body of people for whose sake this duty is carried out. Classic examples of civic duty include paying one's taxes; abiding the law; registering to vote; acting to make sure the voices of all citizens are heard; bearing true witness to violators of the law; coming to the aid of people in need; volunteering for public causes and services; serving in the military, particularly at times of demonstrable peril; and donating time, money, or another good for people who need it.

There are some interesting things to note about these examples: (1) in each case, their fulfillment depends on the existence of other people who make that fulfillment meaningful; (2) in many of the examples the failure to follow through is neither illegal nor enforceably punishable; (3) the motivation for a giver to follow through on the good deed depends on some prior belief in the worthiness of a beneficiary; and, often (4) the performance of the deed hinges on one's belief that one is not alone in carrying it out. Taken together, these features suggest that the successfulness of campaigns launched from the motive of civic duty will be variable and depend to a large degree on what one thinks of the others alongside of whom one lives.

In terms of organ donation, therefore, public opinion polls matter. Thus to effect change it will matter how seriously we think a problem is, such as how much knowledge we have about the growing waiting list of those suffering from end-stage renal disease. It will matter whether we believe such individuals are at the mercy of the good, voluntary work of others. It will even matter whether enough of us believe in general that we are not a society of curmud-geons and misanthropes but rather a collection of good people, all of whom seek to thrive in the polity created for the flourishing of everyone. Societies with a homogeneous demographical makeup may have fewer handicaps to overcome in coming to believe these things, but for all kinds of societies much can be done to engender more buy-in than currently exists across the board, starting with good education campaigns. Without this buy-in, civic duty will not be a powerful impetus for change.

In *The Antichrist* Friedrich Nietzsche asks: "What could destroy us more quickly than working, thinking, and feeling without any inner necessity, without any deeply personal choice, without pleasure—as an automaton of 'duty'? This is the very recipe for decadence, even for idiocy."[52] Nietzsche denies the premise of what powers the emergence of willing, living donors. In specific, he assumes that while society is here to help us cosmetically or in situations where we share interests of utility, the genuine desire to act can em-anate only from within, for one's own betterment. If Nietzsche is right about human nature, authentic displays of altruism are a sham and there is nothing to be crowded-out to begin with. The empirical studies that have been con-ducted to test this theory about human nature, however, seem to conclude otherwise. Most biologists and psychologists today concur that we are not isolated selves, only out for ourselves. Rather, we are an "altruistic species" whose limitations on love of the other for the sake of the other can change, depending on the sort of society we collectively habituate.[53] The nature of the envisioned relationship between the individual and society, and between self-regarding impulses and altruistic ones, can be better understood by looking more closely at actual living organ donors and what they have to say in their own words about the sacrifices they undergo for those who need their help.

NOTES

1. M. Hashem Pesaran, "Econometrics," in *Econometrics: The New Palgrave,* ed. J. Eatwell et al. (New York: Palgrave Macmillan, 1990), 1. Economist Ragnar Frisch is given credit for the sense in which the term "econometrics" is typically employed today, but the term was first used by Polish economist Pawel Ciompa in 1910.

2. Milton Friedman, *Essays in Positive Economics* (Chicago: University of Chicago Press, 1953), 15, 22.

3. As a scholar in the humanities, it is with some trepidation that I travel further into the terrain of the social sciences. I must thank my colleagues in the Program

in Public Health at Stony Brook University for alerting me to the methodologies typically employed in the social sciences for best studying these questions, as well as for directing me to the resources that helped me understand them. I am particularly grateful for the insights and helpful suggestions of Jaymie Meliker, Amy Hammock, Lisa Benzscott, Rachel Kidman, Sean Clouston, Tia Palermo, and Lauren Hale.

4. Amy Friedman, remarks delivered at The Case For and Against the Selling of Organs Conference, Stony Brook University, April 16, 2012. For details about topics and panelists, see: http://www.stonybrook.edu/bioethics/OrganDonorConference Poster.pdf.

5. A. D. Waterman, S. L. Stanley, T. Covelli, E. Hazel, B. A. Hong, and D. C. Brennan, "Living Donation Decision Making: Recipients' Concerns and Educational Needs," *Prog Transplant* 16, no. 4 (2006): 17–23.

6. Katrina A. Bramstedt and Rena Down, *The Organ Donor Experience* (New York: Roman and Littlefield, 2011), 154, 160.

7. Richard Titmuss, *The Gift Relationship: From Human Blood to Social Policy* (New York: Vintage, 1971).

8. Ibid., 267–74.

9. Bruno S. Frey, Felix Oberholzer-Gee, and Reiner Eichenberger, "The Old Lady Visits Your Backyard: A Tale of Morals and Markets," *Journal of Political Economy* 104, no. 6 (1996): 1302.

10. As reported by the International Atomic Energy Agency. See the agency's statistics for nuclear share of electricity for the year 2015 at: https://www.iaea.org/PRIS /WorldStatistics/NuclearShareofElectricityGeneration.aspx.

11. Frey et al., "Old Lady Visits Your Backyard," 1302–3.

12. Bruno Frey and Felix Oberholzer-Gee, "The Cost of Price Incentives: An Empirical Analysis of Crowding-Out," *American Economic Review* 87, no. 4 (1997): 749.

13. Ibid., 749–50, italics in original.

14. Ibid., 749n8.

15. Ibid., 750.

16. Ibid.

17. Ibid.

18. Ibid.

19. The crowding-out thesis, as it applies to organ donation, is not accepted by everyone working on the problem. One critic is Scott Halpern, who argues that the burden ought to be placed on the one who is predicting or speculating about the thesis's plausibility to furnish evidence for his or her case, not the reverse. See Scott D. Halpern, "Regulated Payments for Living Kidney Donation: An Empirical Assessment of the Ethical Concerns," *Annals of Internal Medicine* 152, no. 6 (March 2010): 358–66. In his own study of what people said they *thought* they would do given the inducement of monetary incentives, Halpern found that such an offer would make no difference on a prospective donor's decision to donate. This is a different question than what donors *did* do when offered such an incentive (which is untested due to its illegality). This noted, Halpern's was the only such study I encountered to arrive

at this neutral conclusion. Additionally, Halpern's study fails to take into account what the results would be of offering cash incentives following a robust educational campaign in service of, while removing existing *disincentives* for, donating out of the motive of civic duty along the lines suggested. I must thank Anne Barnhill for calling my attention to Halpern's argument and for additionally pointing out in her own voice that another possible objection is that even if we grant that the crowding-out thesis is true, it behooves us to specify how many individuals would in fact be crowded out. If this number could be made up for by additional individuals who would be recruited by virtue of financial inducements, then this is a consideration that needs to be pragmatically calculated. Again, my belief is that human beings are malleable and cannot be segregated into two classes of responsive donors: those who are positively persuaded by financial incentives and those who are not. The culture and public context make the decisive difference; someone could be one sort of person in one environment and another sort in a different one. Indeed, that is the point.

20. Frey et. al., "Old Lady Visits Your Backyard," 1308.

21. Ibid.

22. Ibid., 1310–11.

23. Michael J. Sandel, *What Money Can't Buy: The Moral Limits of Markets* (New York: Farrar, Straus and Giroux, 2012). See especially chap. 3, "How Markets Crowd Out Morals."

24. Ibid., 98.

25. Ibid., 117–18.

26. Ibid., 118.

27. While the unpaid students collected 55 percent more in donations than those who were offered the lowest financial incentives, they collected only 9 percent more than those on the higher commission. For the original study, see Uri Gneezy and Aldo Rustichini, "Pay Enough or Don't Pay at All," *Quarterly Journal of Economics* 115, no. 3 (August 2000): 799.

28. Granting that there are reasons why we might be inclined to resist the conversion of especially precious goods into cash, one might still wonder if there remains a threshold at which such resistance could be overridden. To be more precise, might there be a point at which so much cash is offered that qualms about civic symbolism give way to real-world opportunities that large amounts of money open up? If such a threshold exists, then isn't this whole debate a matter of resetting the price at which the precious good in question is correctly valued? This is the same sort of response raised by the deregulator who wants the market alone to determine the value of a kidney. Indeed, this might become a solution—everything, as they say, has a price—but at what other costs? Charge too much, we recall, and we have a society in which rich people are walking around with exorbitantly priced body parts taken from the poor. One may do the extrapolation with regard to paying for adopted babies, or surrogates, or so forth. Ultimately the extra gains one receives by pricing a good very high must be weighed against the additional social costs that such pricing brings about.

29. Uri Gneezy and Aldo Rustichini, "A Fine Is a Price," *Journal of Legal Studies* 29, no. 1 (January 2000): 1–17. Discussed by Sandel, *What Money Can't Buy,* 119.

30. Sandel, *What Money Can't Buy*, 119.

31. See, for example, Aristotle, *Nicomachean Ethics*, trans. Terence Irwin, 2nd ed. (Indianapolis, IN: Hackett, 1999), 1103.

32. J. Elster, *Solomonic Judgments: Studies in Limitations of Rationality* (Cambridge: Cambridge University Press, 1989).

33. Bruno Frey, "A Constitution of Knaves Crowds Out Civic Virtues," *Economic Journal* 107, no. 443 (July 1997): 1047–48.

34. Ibid., 1051.

35. Ibid., 1052.

36. L. E. Boulware, M. U. Troll, N. Y. Wang, and N. R. Powe, "Public Attitudes towards Incentives for Organ Donation: A National Study of Different Racial/Ethnic and Income Groups," *American Journal of Transplantation* 6 (2006): 2774–85.

37. Jagbir Gill, James Dong, Caren Rose, Olwyn Johnston, David Landsberg, and John Gill, "The Effect of Race and Income on Living Kidney Donation in the United States," *Journal of the American Society of Nephrology* (2013). See: http://jasn.asnjournals.org/content/early/2013/08/28/ASN.2013010049.full.

38. Ibid.

39. For a good discussion of how race, privilege, and similar factors bear on the extent to which vulnerable communities come to engender distrust in scientific and medical institutions over time, see Rebecca Skloot, *The Immortal Life of Henrietta Lacks* (New York: Random House, 2010).

40. Gill et al., "Effect of Race and Income."

41. Ibid.

42. Nir Eyal et al., "An Open Letter to President Barack Obama, Secretary of Health and Human Services Sylvia Mathews Burwell, Attorney General Eric Holder and Leaders of Congress," September 11, 2014, http://ustransplantopenletter.org/openletter.html.

43. Klaus Hoeyer, Silke Schicktanz, and Ida Deleuran, "Public Attitudes to Financial Incentive Models for Organs: A Literature Review Suggests That It Is Time to Shift the Focus from 'Financial Incentives' to Reciprocity," *Transplant International* 26 (2013): 354.

44. Ibid.

45. Ibid., 355.

46. Ibid., 355–56, italics in original.

47. As reported in my interview with Lauren Muskauski on July 30, 2015. Lauren kept a close diary of her living donation experience and reported the whole process in a nine-part blog. See: http://livinglegacymd.wordpress.com/2012/03/23/my-living-donation-journey-part-1-the-decision/, last accessed June 30, 2016.

48. Boulware et al., "Public Attitudes toward Incentives for Organ Donation," 2774.

49. For a list of these studies, see Amy D. Waterman and James R. Rodrigue, "Ethically and Effectively Advancing Living Donation: How Should It Be Done?," in *Understanding Organ Donation: Applied Behavioral Science Perspectives*, ed. Jason T. Siegel and Eusebio M. Alvaro (Malden, MA: Wiley-Blackwell, 2010), 293.

50. Ibid., 304.

51. Ibid.

52. Friedrich Nietzsche, *The Antichrist* (§11) in *The Portable Nietzsche*, trans. Walter Kaufmann (New York: Penguin, 1954).

53. See Andrew Michael Flescher and Daniel L. Worthen, *The Altruistic Species: Scientific, Philosophical, and Religious Perspectives of Human Benevolence* (Philadelphia: Templeton, 2007), especially chaps. 2 and 3 on biological and psychological approaches.

4

Living Donors and the Confluence of Altruism and Self-Regard

COMPLEX HUMAN MOTIVATIONS AND THE MYTH OF UNMOTIVATED ALTRUISM

To what extent does money really make the world go around? This question, aside from addressing the moral appropriateness and pragmatic effectiveness of financial incentives with which we have up to this point been preoccupied, asks also about who we are as human beings and what makes us tick. What goes through our minds when others press us into their service or, as is often the case with living organ donors, we press ourselves into service? Is this something we do for a hidden, selfish reason? Alternatively, is a planned sacrifice of the magnitude of donating an organ indicative of some superhuman saintliness that is neither common to nor reflective of what motivates most human beings? As a living donor advocate I have come to learn that donors are neither self-satisfiers nor moral paragons. Rather, they are ordinary individuals who simultaneously want to help someone else and fulfill their own need to forge a connection with someone or deepen an already existing one. Living donors demonstrate that human beings are at once self-regarding and altruistic. They are ready to sacrifice for others not for a singular reason but because of a number of factors that, surprisingly, turn out to be compatible with one another.

Some skeptics wonder if such thing as "pure" or "unmotivated" altruism even exists. They maintain that self-sacrificial giving to others is reducible to self-interest at a further remove: in the end *some* pay-off (even if it is the avoidance of something unpleasant) accounts for most people's decisions to help others. Altruism is apparent but not genuine. If this is true, it follows that directly providing financial incentives to living donors is both the most honest and the most efficient means of attending to the needs of those

111

seeking organs. Others maintain that such a thing as acting for the other's sake is real but that *only* by taking action in this manner will we know that we have averted the corrupting influence of self-interest. As Immanuel Kant proposed, we know that we have done right only if we have removed any self-regarding pay-off from the course of action we are considering.[1] In the case of donating organs, this would mean that only by forgoing a large payment of money and also by not receiving future healthcare benefits can we be sure that we have acted rightly.

Positing a contrast between altruism and self-regard is, however, to promote a false dichotomy. First of all, receiving a measured form of compensation like long-term health care in order to remove disincentives to donating is not only an efficient approach, it is not morally problematic in the same way that offering a lump sum of money is. More important, however, are the self-regarding needs that the altruistic gesture of donating an organ fulfills for the giver. What we must consider is whether altruistic and self-regarding impulses can coexist in a symbiotic relationship, where altruism is understood to be a shared activity. On this account, donating one's organs is tantamount to acting in a way that is bereft of egoistic motive. This noted, the fulfilling nature of the act of sacrifice is usually not without qualification. Almost without exception, the prospective donors whose comments provide the basis for this argument expressed a desire to get to know their recipients personally or, if they knew them already, to get to know them better, or differently. While they report that moving forward with the donation is not, strictly speaking, conditional on deepening this connection with their recipient—and are nevertheless still willing to step forward as donors—remaining dispassionately at an arm's distance is not their preference.

This understanding of altruism as a shared activity is consistent with the insights of C. Daniel Batson, who argues that selfless behavior is not reducible to a particular motive or set of outcomes in which the benefits flow in one direction only. Indirect or proximate benefits may accrue for the giver without impugning his or her original good and other-regarding intent. Batson's "empathy-altruism" hypothesis allows both the giver and the recipient to benefit from a noble sacrificial act and also for the giver to take pleasure in the giving.[2] According to Batson, over the course of our evolutionary history our ability to empathize with those who need our help has produced long-term adaptively advantageous outcomes for rendering this help.[3] The empathy-altruism hypothesis implies that our capacity to identify with the woes of others is a naturally occurring phenomenon in human nature that leads us to help them prior to any consideration of forthcoming reward. It need not be spurred by external incentives. Prosocial motivation is not a ploy but a genuine internal process that exists alongside other basic material and psychological needs.

Of course, just because altruistic motivation is genuine does not preclude the fact that there is a range within which it naturally occurs in human experience. Batson does not deny that altruistic motivation is subject to pressure and limitation. The pull of special relationships or unusual hardship, for example, may restrict an individual's capacity to extend his or her "circle of concern." Not everyone will have the resources, the good timing, or the ability to cultivate the disposition to do something as selflessly impactful as donating an organ. But when one is able to rise to such an occasion, one does so not departing from the evolutionary constraints that limit human selflessness but rather as a fully adjusted human being coming into one's own. If Batson is right, then it might be perfectly rational, even healthy, to undergo voluntarily a procedure not in one's own best immediate medical interests but which ends up serving one's long-term welfare and well-being. Having this ambition for its own sake does not make you a masochist or a person suffering from some psychological disorder.[4] Nor does it make you a self-denying saint. Giving something so precious as a bodily organ, and giving it for the ultimate sake of the one in need, additionally affords the giver the pleasurable and meaningful benefit of having participated in a profoundly sharing and community-building activity.

Philosophers in the Aristotelian tradition concur that in a broader sense, selfless forms of virtue are an integral part of self-regard. As Jean Hampton notes, to love another fully should not entail relinquishing all sense of one's personhood. "Self-sacrifice cannot be commendable if it springs from self-abnegation. . . . If we are so 'altruistic' that we become unable to develop and express ourselves properly, we become unable to give to others what they may want more than anything else."[5] Aristotle himself puts the point in a positive light in the *Nicomachean Ethics*: "When everyone competes to achieve what is fine and strains to do the finest actions, everything that is right will be done for the common good, and each person will receive the greatest of goods, since that is the character of virtue. Hence, the good person must be a self-lover, since he will both help himself and benefit others by doing fine actions."[6] As Aristotle observes, our character development furnishes us with the requisite virtue for other-regard, which in turn amplifies the prospects for our own participation in the good.

Aristotle was prescient. The science explaining not just the psychological advantages but also the other health benefits of engaging in significant helping behaviors is today sprouting into a substantial and growing discipline, so much so that we now know something about how the costs borne of sacrificing for others can be offset by hormonal and even cardiovascular benefits.[7] While most living donors are not aware of these benefits, they do tend to feel and often are even able to articulate their sense of the benefit to themselves for what they are about to do. Donors consistently express similar reasoning by which they have autonomously planned, without coercion, to donate an organ for someone else who needs it. They deny that donating the organ is something to be regarded as "above and beyond"—according to them they have no real choice but to act for the sake of the one(s) they love—and they look forward to their near futures with genuine enthusiasm and anticipation. One of the most critical responsibilities of the living donor advocate is to be able to distinguish whether this sense of inner compulsion emanates from an external or outward coercion, the presence of which disqualifies a prospective donor from following through on his or her stated intentions. This entails being able to discern true self-awareness of the donor.

How is one to become confident that the one sacrificing knows what he or she is doing and is doing that thing for the right reasons? Granting, for the sake of argument (and in temporary agreement with the skeptic) that there is technically no such thing as "unmotivated" altruism—that is, some pure form of other-regard or sacrifice undertaken without any ambition or even expectation of self-regarding implications—is it reasonably possible to distinguish the sort of giving that is healthy and within the realm of ordinary human experience from the sort that is pathological or otherwise forced? For some guidance, it may be helpful to take a look at some controversial kidney donation cases in order to ascertain a better understanding of how donors perceive their altruistic sacrifice in their own terms.

LIVING DONORS AND LIVING DONOR ADVOCACY

One of the main arguments in favor of legalizing the sale of organs is that it is unfair to take advantage of the good graces of the living donor, who makes an enormous sacrifice and accrues no benefits to himself or herself, while others, including the medical staff and recipient, do benefit. This view assumes that altruism is a sucker's bet and not the move of the savvy player. If, however, human beings are hardwired to be altruistic and to better themselves as they better others, the need to protect irrational self-abnegators who somehow do not protect themselves becomes less pressing. In this case, there would be no need for financial reward: a different and more organic form of compensation, inherent in the giving process itself, is already fulfilling the needs of the giver, who is not being exploited.

The presence of such a motivation, however, cannot be assumed. It is crucial that living donor advocates are reliably able to rule out the presence of coercive factors to stop donation by people who are not competent to freely or rationally decide on their own behalf. Coercive factors run the gamut and include any familial or cultural pressure exerted on the donor to undergo a transplantation; any demonstrable mental incapacity or defect that would compromise the donor's decision-making capacity; any imbalance in the relationship between the donor and the recipient (for example, feelings of guilt or blinding romantic affection or fear on the part of the donor); or any promise of financial or other reward, the offer of which is not only illegal but also raises the possibility that the donor would not have chosen to donate without the promise of such a reward. The presence of any one of these factors is a red flag that should make the attentive living donor advocate worry that the donor is not in a position to make a fully voluntary decision of such magnitude.

Even so, the decision to donate is often easy to understand and concerns about coercion can be ruled out quickly. Most donors are either family members by blood who are close in age to their recipients or spouses or partners who fortunately happen to be a match for their loved one. In these cases the confluence of altruism and self-regard is readily apparent. Not only is the recipient among the select group of people within the donor's circle of concern, but these relationships are usually uncomplicated: the two individuals love each other dearly and know that if the roles were reversed the recipient would act in kind. It is not uncommon to hear donors say that it is a blessing to be able to give a kidney to the one they love. These living donors are the majority, and most of the advocate's time is spent in reminding the donor of what the procedure will be like and other details related to it (like how much time they must take off from work or how little weight they will be able to carry for the forthcoming weeks).

Occasionally, however, the donor and recipient are not part of each other's regular life or, if they are, they have only recently become so or the two interact in a way that involves some other unusual qualifier. When this occurs, it is incumbent on the donor advocate to pay close attention during the interview and ask the right questions in order to successfully elicit evidence that the donor is fully informed and willing while also not unnecessarily discouraging the donor from carrying through on his or her intentions.

We can learn a great deal about donor motivation by reflecting on living donors who donate to more-distant recipients, whether they are not that close to or have not known the recipient for a long time, or even if they are complete strangers. These donors often come across as cogent and stable people with more than the average amount of coherence and conviction to explain both the chronology of and reasoning for their decision. They know better than the libertarian or transplant surgeon whether the offer of a substantial amount of money would have made any difference in their decision. In order to get a better understanding of the confluence of altruism and self-regard that inheres in donor motivation, a review of three cases will be helpful. (The names of the donors and recipients involved have all been changed.)[8]

A. THE EX-SPOUSE

May 20th, 2015

Dear Steve:

On Friday, May 22nd, I met with Robert Richards (59 years old), who plans to donate his kidney to his ex-wife, Sally Richards. At the moment, surgery is booked for 6/16/2015, timed for when Mr. Richards's school year ends (he teaches health education to middle-school students), but the operation is now pending the results of a cat scan to follow up on nodules detected on his lung. Mr. Richards, who lives in California, plans to have this testing done this week.

I discussed at length with Mr. Richards the unusual circumstance of one deciding to donate to one's ex-spouse, and we spoke in particular about what led him to this decision. Mr. Richards impressed upon me that this was not a flippant, sudden, or emotional decision, but rather one he'd put more than a year's thought into and one about which he'd never wavered. When I asked him specifically what led to the decision, Mr. Richards replied: "If more of us would see people on dialysis, we'd know this is something we should do if we are in a position to be able to do it." Mr. Richards articulated that despite that he was often not able to get along with his ex-wife when they were married, or on occasion even now in conversation, he loved her and was resolute that this was what he wanted to do. He did intimate that he wasn't the best husband. He was the one in the marriage who'd often "failed to follow through." But he also insisted that donating his kidney was not some gesture to atone for any past sins, but rather a "no-brainer" based on the opportunity he was given to help someone he cared so much about.

I explained to Mr. Richards about what the process of donating would be, what the risks were, and that this was not something that was necessarily in his own best medical interests. He understood everything completely. I explained to him what it means that I am his advocate and he knows I am an independent entity there for him. He has my cell phone number and I instructed him to call me at any time for any reason.

The one area of concern I had going into this interview was that Mr. Richards had not planned to bring a family member or friend to be with him the first week following surgery. He has scheduled for his mother to be here, but only up until the day of surgery. I impressed upon him how important it is that he have someone he trusts and who loves him nearby to help him carry things and attend to the routine tasks of daily life as well as to monitor him for potential (even if unlikely) complications immediately after the operation. By the end of the conversation he seemed convinced that he needed to bring someone with him and promised me he would.

At this time, I have no concerns. I believe that Mr. Richards is fully informed and freely consenting in his decision to donate his kidney to his former wife.

Sincerely,
Andrew Flescher
Living Donor Advocate

B. MET ON FACEBOOK

June 1st, 2015

Dear Steve:

Today I met with Eileen Cooper (27 years old), who is scheduled in August to donate a kidney to Mary Saudino (19 years old). In general, I found Ms. Cooper's reflections about the wonderful thing she is about to do affirm the assessment provided on her work-up by her psychologist, Karen O'Sullivan. Ms. Cooper is fully informed and doing this for the following reasons, each consistent with one another: (1) to help someone in need; (2) to forge bonds with the "donate for life" community; (3) because she herself almost died when she was four years old and, by her reckoning, was given terrific treatment at Stony Brook Hospital twenty-three years ago. She mentioned she wants to give back to her community and "pay it forward." She is informed about the risks involved in her upcoming nephrectomy, and knows that there is no medical benefit to her for giving her kidney. She became aware of Mary Saudino's plight, as many did, on Facebook, where Mary has for the last month publicly sought a volunteer. As Ms. Cooper put it to Karen O'Sullivan and to us, she sees her decision as following through on an idea "that has always existed in the back of my mind." There is no question she understands what she is about to do, what disruption it will mean in the short term to her work and comfort level, and what medical issues might surface in the long run, despite their low risk. She is in perfect health and understands this makes her not only a good candidate to donate in terms of the longevity of the graft but also in terms of her own well-being post-op.

Because this is a case of an altruistic donor, I asked Ms. Cooper to consider some hypotheticals which I do not always bring up in advocacy meetings. In this conversation I had to balance competing considerations:

(1) I wanted to make sure I informed the donor about the context of her giving this gift (which comes at a cost to her), so that her consent was genuine.

(2) I wanted to make sure to phrase things hypothetically so as to respect the privacy of the recipient's family and so as to not violate HIPAA.

(3) I wanted to make sure not to dissuade the donor from retaining the generous spirit she has engendered going into this process.

I asked Ms. Cooper to think about what it would be like if it turned out Mary Saudino was taciturn or not socially comfortable connecting with her, thus impeding the possibility that they'd become close or that her family could become close to the recipient's family. Would this affect her decision? Ms. Cooper admitted that while this wouldn't be her preference, she would still go through with it. (She was resolute in expressing this.) I then explained to her that once she donated her kidney—indeed once anybody does—the recipient is the steward of this gift and it is no longer within the donor's control as to what happens to it. Hypothetically, Mary Saudino could abuse alcohol and drugs and ruin the kidney Ms. Cooper gives her. Ms. Cooper understood this possibility and had already reflected on it. Finally, I broached the thorny issue—again, as a hypothetical (despite that it is a true detail of this case and one that has given all of us concern): it could be that the recipient has a sibling who is a perfect match, but for whatever reason that sibling is not available as a donor. (I did not reveal that Mary Saudino's mother has been adamant with us that both of her daughters not be under anesthesia at the same time and for this reason has ruled out her other daughter as a donor to her sister.) Would it bother Ms. Cooper, in this scenario, again presented hypothetically, that the recipient was waiting to see if an altruistic donor might step forward before she asked her own sister to consider donating? To further distance this hypothetical from the truth of the matter, I intimated to Ms. Cooper that I sometimes ask these same questions to other prospective kidney donors. This last hypothetical, unlike the previous ones I'd raised, did make Ms. Cooper pause and think. After a couple of moments, however, she repeated to me that donating this kidney was what she wanted to do to and that she was aware of what she was doing.

Ms. Cooper then expressed that she was thankful I'd been so candid. She may have gotten a clue that I was raising the hypothetical to alert her to a real possibility, but she didn't probe further. She knows that I am available to her 24/7 to talk about anything for whatever reason. She has my personal cell phone number and knows to contact me if she has any questions prior to the procurement scheduled for mid-August. Despite Mary Saudino's initial reticence to Ms. Cooper's proposal that both families meet, she eventually agreed, and we are now in the process of setting up a breakfast where the donor and recipient and their families can break bread with each other and exchange pleasantries.

Sincerely,

Andrew Flescher

Living Donor Advocate

IT'S A MATCH!

January 20th, 2016

Dear Steve:

This morning I met with Lisa Igler, age 22, and her mother, Deborah, in the capacity as her living donor advocate. Lisa is scheduled to donate her kidney to her girlfriend, Ariana Dorado, on Tuesday, February 2nd, 2016, whom she has been dating since August, 2015. Lisa currently works two jobs, both of which require significant physical activity and readiness: she coaches cheerleaders and she works with severely disturbed and often mentally handicapped individuals in a home. Lisa's blood type is O positive, the same type as her girlfriend, Ariana. Without immediately involving Ariana in her investigation into whether she would be a suitable match to donate her kidney, Lisa carefully gathered information and became an informed prospective donor. I haven't a doubt that this is what Lisa wants to do, that she wasn't coerced by her girlfriend, and that her parents, who might have been initially skeptical, have themselves come to embrace Lisa's plan to give the gift of life, as they trust their daughter's judgment as well as the good character of her girlfriend, the recipient. I came to this conclusion after an hour discussion with Lisa and her mother. Although she has a history of ADHD, and has been on medication for it prescribed by her psychiatrist in Maryland, Lisa is otherwise healthy. She has been seen and cleared both by Dr. Heesuck Suh and by her own psychiatrist.

A little background: Lisa is a registered plasma donor, has worked with the Red Cross to coordinate blood donation, and had done a significant amount of thinking about what it means to be a blood, plasma, or organ donor, all long before she met Ariana. Getting to know Ariana, Lisa learned she suffered from Lupus. She saw Ariana go through a hospitalization in September, which is when she first learned Ariana needed a kidney and started to think seriously about being Ariana's donor. It was then when Lisa learned that Ariana needed peritoneal dialysis every night, and, Lisa explained to me, when she became acquainted up close with what it was like for an individual to live one's life dependent on dialysis. Upon querying her specifically, Lisa told me that it was exclusively her idea to become a donor for Ariana. Lisa notified Ariana's physician that she was seriously contemplating becoming a donor for her, asked a few more questions, and got tested to see if she would be suitable. She then made up her mind a couple weeks later and surprised Ariana with a gift, as depicted in the attached You Tube video, which, upon going viral overnight, was picked up by Inside Edition, which featured their story this past week.

Since then Lisa has been contacted by producers of MTV's Real World, among other program producers, to publicize the story of her and Ariana, whom she first met on the romantic online dating site Tinder. I was impressed with Lisa's unwavering conviction that she would at no point accept any money for her potential involvement with these programs. If money were to come from participating in offers to capture their story, it would be directed to some foundation sympathetic to the cause of organ transplantation. I was also impressed with the clarity and resolve with which Lisa expressed that she knew for sure that this is what she wanted to do. I specifically asked her (and her mother revealed she too had previously asked her daughter) whether hearing from these television shows put any additional pressure on her to follow through with her intentions. She expressed, convincingly, that it had no bearing.

I answered questions Lisa and her mother had about follow-up appointments post-op, informed them of the several things she needed to be aware of immediately after surgery (e.g., no more ibuprofen; no lifting anything more than ten pounds for a few weeks; no working for six weeks) and gave my cell phone number where I could be reached 24/7. I am confident that donating her kidney to Ariana is something Lisa freely desires to do and that she is informed about her so doing. I told Lisa that I or someone would visit her on 17 North at Stony Brook Hospital on February 3rd to see how she did.

Sincerely,

Andrew Flescher

Living Donor Advocate

COMMENTARY

These three examples ask us to determine whether or not the sacrifice the donor is poised to make is voluntary, informed, and something that puts neither the donor's safety nor his or her autonomy in any kind of jeopardy. In the first case, it is reasonable to wonder whether the ex-husband might be motivated by guilt as a result of a failed marriage in which he was the one, by his own reckoning, who had let his wife down when they were together. In the second case was there an obligation to reveal the true context in which the donor was preparing to give her kidney to a stranger she'd met on Facebook? Was it her right to know that the recipient also had a sister near in age who was a perfect match but who was deemed unavailable by the recipient's mother? Perhaps by knowing this she'd have had a clearer understanding of why the recipient was initially reluctant to have the families meet. In the third case, it was only a few weeks after the two individuals met through an online dating site when one of the women made a decision to give her kidney to the other. Was this too soon? At the age of twenty-two, was she too young to make such a weighty choice? Had the recipient subconsciously or seductively exerted any pressure on the donor to sacrifice for her sake? Conversely, if the nature of the relationship were to change or end, would following through on this decision make the recipient permanently beholden to the donor in some inappropriate manner?

Behind all of these questions is the common question about what incentivizes people to make a major gift to a new acquaintance, to a stranger, or, as in the first case, to one to whom one has become estranged. What are the expectations these donors have of their recipients, and does the fact that donors might *have* expectations impugn their giving act? It is crucial that donor advocates rule out the existence of incentives that suggest undue pressure on a living donor. In allowing a transplantation to proceed, advocates must be able to sense that donors continue to remain their normal selves and certainly that they are not preparing themselves for the role of self-abnegator.

This being said, donors tend to be aware that they are about to undergo major surgery that they don't medically need. But they are undergoing surgery for a reason, one which often has something to do with the relationship they hope to encourage between themselves and their recipients. On rare occasions this affective component is not detected; its absence signals a red flag. For example, a donor who steps forward on the basis of a utilitarian calculation, with no perceptible emotional interest on his or her part in the recipient, causes concern.[9] This rarely happens, however. The more common situation in cases of "altruistic" donation—that is, donations between strangers—occurs when the donor admits he or she wants something back from the recipient.

This "something" is not money. Rather, it is acknowledgment, appreciation, and the desire to become a different, better person. The less-than-dependable former husband, Robert, expressed his wish to volunteer for his ex-wife, Sally, not to absolve himself from lingering remorse but rather to experience the joy he failed to absorb fully while married: of being able to be available for someone else who needed what he, uniquely, had to offer. Eileen responded open-heartedly to Mary's Facebook appeal because of a memory that had stayed with her throughout her life of being saved as a child at the same hospital now giving her the opportunity to pay it forward. After all those years, she still saw herself as an integral part of the Stony Brook community and believed, in offering her kidney to Mary, that she was doing her part to strengthen this community further. Lisa, it is true, had fallen in love with Ariana by the time she'd decided to give Ariana her kidney, but it was evident that she'd spent a considerable amount of time prior to meeting Ariana in building up to this moment of donation. She was a plasma donor and had worked with the Red Cross coordinating nationwide blood donation efforts. Donating an organ, she explained, had always been something she was seriously considering. She'd been waiting for the right situation to present itself. Her decision to donate a kidney was not encouraged by the recipient. To the contrary, it germinated from within Lisa herself as the natural next step in her development into the kind of woman she wanted to become. These cases reinforce the notion that donating a kidney represents a priceless opportunity for the giver to mature into the sort of person who is a lover of humanity and the common good. None of the donors were missing self-regarding motivation, but their motivation stemmed from a desire to help someone else and had a more powerful and visceral grip on them than the prospect of financial remuneration.

Two of these three planned nephrectomies, in the end, did not go through. A health risk surfaced for one at the eleventh hour, and a kidney stone appeared just days before the second was scheduled to be operated on. A team consisting of the transplant surgeon, the living donor coordinator, and the living donor advocate concluded that the risks involved in moving forward would be unacceptably high. Not surprisingly, the two individuals who were not able to donate expressed considerable dismay that in the end they weren't in the position to follow through on their plans, although in both cases they participated productively in the discussions that led to their eventually backing out. Nevertheless, all three examples affirm that the process worked as it was supposed to work, with responsible third parties looking out for the interests of the donors even as the donors themselves sought to be available for a recipient. That no financial contract between donor and recipient hung in the balance made it easier when the time came to change course. No one had to worry about whether a pending monetary transaction would put added pressure on donors to proceed with the nephrectomies, which could have been unsafe. All three examples jointly affirm Batson's empathy-altruism hypothesis: by carefully distinguishing the perspectives of all actors and recipients, there is room to preserve the interests of everyone involved. Altruism does not flow in one direction from giver to recipient, from saint to sufferer.

On the contrary, altruism is a shared activity not enshrouded in the rarified air of martyrdom but upheld in sensible, community-enhancing policies designed to bolster trust in the system. This observation is consistent with the ethnographic work Katrina A. Bramstedt and Rena Down have done by examining and reporting on altruistic living donors. As they note, the ambition to sacrifice for others is not an inducement for donors to take leave of their senses. For donors it is empathy, the understanding and identifying with the feelings of another, that grounds the urge to donate. Empathy, as Bramstedt and Down describe it, is a concept conveying "interconnection." They characterize it this way because "another" is a "neighbor" just as humanity belongs to "one family."[10] According to this view, the giver is able to see in the recipient the common plight of the one struggling against misfortune even as misfortune manifests itself differently in each sufferer.

Empathy entails not a hierarchical ordering between giver and recipient in which the former elevates himself or herself above the one he or she is preparing to save. It is a "prosocial act" in which the giver sees himself or herself in the recipient.[11] Bramstedt and Down locate in the giver four aspects of empathy: perspective taking (defined as "the donor's spontaneous attempts to adopt the perspectives of others and see things from their point of view"); fantasy (the ability for the donor to imaginatively adopt this perspective); empathic concern (warmth, compassion, and other sentimental states that impel other-regarding action); and personal distress (a donor's feeling of negativity as he or she witnesses the suffering of the future recipient).[12] These aspects of empathy are both cognitive and emotional.[13] They lead to compassionate action because of the deliberate and concrete movement of understanding and intimacy one person takes in the direction of another. Interviews reveal the critical role that bridging the initial distance between giver and recipient plays in the donor's ability to engender empathy.

The intimacy created in the process is nonnegotiable. In theory, utilitarianism, an ideology entailing widespread buy-in to the principle of the greatest good for the greatest number, could lead to a world in which we all came to mutually see the benefits of offering our own bodies as potential sources for organs. In practice, however, there is no circumventing the emotional component in which donors come to believe in reasons that relate to their own biographies for understanding and caring about others. Empathy, in other words, is not self-generated; it is other-oriented.[14]

Thus a giver's gift is not independent of but is ironically contingent on the other's acknowledgment and receipt of it. Gift-giving is a profoundly relational act, one involving connection and trust. Trust does not occur in a vacuum or exist as a resource of which one can privately avail oneself. By contrast, it is

> linked to neighborliness and altruism. This is because trust cannot occur in isolation but rather involves *another* party (neighbor). In its form as a noun, the word "trust" involves taking on responsibility for someone (or something), as in trusteeship. As a verb, "trust" involves having faith or confidence in a person or a thing. Personality psychologists have studied these concepts and determined that we tend to feel responsible for people we trust and tend to feel bad when they experience problems originating without their control (illness). Trusting people are also more likely to give these individuals helpful services. In the setting of organ donation, these

are the neighbors whom Good Samaritans respond to when hearing about or seeing their affliction, especially those cases involving childhood genetic disorders such as cystic fibrosis and biliary atresia.[15]

If empathy is conceptually linked to trust in this manner, then the giver is not only not hierarchically superior to the recipient in the giving process; he or she is also, importantly, vulnerable to the recipient. This conclusion is borne out in the three cases described above. An ex-husband, a perfect stranger prior to a chance encounter on Facebook, and a partner in a budding romantic relationship, each for their own idiosyncratic reasons, saw in their giving act the chance to become better people. However, to become better people, they were at the mercy of their recipients' willingness to accept and be grateful for their pending Good Samaritanism. A too-casual acknowledgment on the part of the recipient of the donor's gesture might have discouraged the donor, if not jeopardized the planned gift entirely.

The enthusiasm with which donors gear up to sacrifice for others, in other words, seems conditional on the expectation of furthering a relationship between the giver and the recipient, even if that relationship does not necessarily flourish following the donation. The hope that it will flourish is what brings the donor forward. This is so even when donors and recipients begin as strangers. Rejected on this account of altruism in donor motivation is the notion of the giver as the self-contained, superhuman hero whose actions spring exclusively from within the resource base of the self. Sacrifice is not a grandiose gesture to be celebrated in the abstract. It is an up-close, communal encounter with a replenishing character. Altruistic sacrifices are remembered and, when a new opportunity arises, paid forward. Their costs entail benefits, and these benefits spur future sacrificial acts.

Bramstedt and Down's research also underscores a theme that has recurred in our discussion thus far: the non-anonymous nature of giving. In almost every case on which they reported, donors got to know their recipients, whether before the transplantation or shortly after. For the few donors who did not get to do so, the missing experience took its toll. One donor complained of a "false hope" given to her by the transplant center, which she felt had promised her that she eventually would meet her recipient. Another, who was told in advance that he would not be able to meet his recipient as a condition of the transplantation being allowed to occur, nevertheless felt "he should, at a minimum, be privy to medical and quality-of-life updates about the clinical status of his organ recipient."[16] In no case reported by Bramstedt and Down, nor any of my own, has a living donor been perfectly okay with not getting to know something about the person who received the organ. Indeed, it is hard to imagine any instance of living donor transplantation in which donors would somehow lose this curiosity or, for that matter, reconcile it with a system in which they were paid for their donation.

The donor-recipient encounter seems to be more native to the overall health of the exchange than any offer of money could successfully eliminate. Most living donors who do get to know their recipients (with permission) follow their recipients' progress, acutely feeling distress in those instances where the graft fails to take or where the recipient becomes gravely sick because of complications or other reasons.[17] The norm is for donors and recipients to stay in touch with one another for the remainder of their lives. Again, it is hard to imagine how this relationship could be severed, or made any less entangled, with the introduction of money, despite all we have seen about how the introduction of money could negatively bear on the relationship. The bond between donors and recipients is one of the strongest that exists between two people; it is created prior to discussions about how the exchange of organs is to take place. Trust between the two parties is presumed. That trust can be damaged, but it cannot be removed from the exchange, whether or not we tinker with the system of compensation.

THE HEALTH BENEFITS OF LIVING DONATION

Living donation has been taking place since 1954, with well over 100,000 people to date having given a kidney or a partial lobe of their liver. Roughly between 5,000 and 6,000 people annually are living donors, which on average amounts to between 20 and 30 percent of all organ transplantations carried out in a year.[18] While these numbers could be higher, they are significant enough that we now have reliable data on some of the health benefits for living donors. The risk of death during a nephrectomy is 3 in 10,000, well within the acceptable risk level for elective surgery. For the large majority of donors, the remaining kidney works fine for the remainder of their life, coming to assume, over time, 70 percent of the function that both kidneys had accounted for together prior to surgery. Kidney donors are no more likely than nondonors to get kidney disease, much less renal failure, after donating (less than 1 percent). While it still remains to be seen whether a nephrectomy makes living donors more susceptible to type 2 diabetes ten or more years down the line, if this or any other long-term consequence leads to kidney failure, the living donor goes to the very top of the waiting list for a kidney transplant (with the exception of two rare situations that take precedence).[19] Besides these potential costs, however, there are considerable health and psychological benefits that the living donor experiences, both acutely and over time.

Multiple studies show that living-related renal donors and altruistic donors alike do not express regret following donation, but these individuals also report enhanced self-esteem.[20] In a study conducted of almost a thousand living donors, E. M. Johnson and colleagues report that the large majority of them reported "excellent quality of life" post-nephrectomy, scoring higher as a group than the national norm on the SF-36, a standardized quality-of-life health questionnaire.[21] Longer-term benefits accruing to living donors have also been well-documented, including increase in self-esteem as a result of receiving regular praise and recognition, weight loss, increased self-awareness about health and mortality, optimized work-life balance and whole-person care, and an inner satisfaction for doing good.[22]

Moving beyond the health benefits of altruism in the narrow cases of living organ donation, many more studies have demonstrated the association, and in some instances causation between grand gestures of altruism and quality of life. There is now ample evidence that significantly selfless behaviors enhance longevity due to the chemicals released in the body that boost immunity and lessen stress.[23] Two of these are oxytocin, a neurotransmitter that is released centrally by the pituitary gland that has been demonstrated to amplify our capacity to trust and feel empathy for the plight of others; and progesterone, a hormone whose level increases in response to forming bonds with others and is related to the desire to put the interests of others above our own.[24]

Health psychologists Stephanie Brown and Michael Brown have proposed a caregiving model based on the regulatory functions of the human neuro-hormonal system, which has evolved over time to facilitate maternal care. The model describes the causal mechanism between altruistic or prosocial behavior and health and longevity. As they explain in somewhat technical detail, the release of hormones that regulate helping behaviors, "governed by the medial preoptic area of the hypothalamus, interacting with certain other brain regions . . . and neuromodulators (especially oxytocin and progesterone)," function in the body by offering stress-buffering and restorative properties, thereby establishing the link between helping others and positive health outcomes.[25] Based on Allan Luks's survey of thousands of volunteers across the nation, he and Peggy Payne have described a "helper's high" that begins with a warm aura marked by the release of endorphins throughout the body that continues as longer-lasting feelings of equanimity and stable, communally oriented living.[26]

Donors' testimonials about their own transplantation experiences often reveal powerful feelings of happiness and life satisfaction that we would be hard-pressed to imagine as present in comparable self-evaluations following the experience of being paid for services. These mental and physical health benefits together serve as grounds for questioning the commonsensical notion that only a financial incentive can adequately convince donors to proceed with the great sacrifice they are poised to make.

There is, no doubt, another side to the story. In addition to these health benefits and reports of increase in happiness, occasionally donors complain of the opposite. In one study from Sweden, for example, 28 percent of individuals interviewed reported feeling "abandoned and exploited."[27] These "minority reports" should come as no surprise, as no two people are alike and any course or path that carries risk will manifest itself variously in terms of costs borne among the pool of risk-takers. That being said, these negative testimonials do not compare with the negative ones that have surfaced among paid living donors in parts of the world where the practice once was legal (primarily India; see chapter 2). Still, negative reports do call attention to the need for compensatory measures to offset the hardships, financial and otherwise, that living donors often experience post-donation, even when those hardships merely take the form of a letdown following the emotional event of a nephrectomy.

Finally, beyond the subjective experience of the giver, and returning to the pragmatic problem of what will work in terms of reducing the organ shortage gap, there is also evidence beginning to surface about a "domino effect" related to becoming a living donor. When one learns of another living donor, one is more likely to become a donor as well; and once one has become a living donor, one is also more likely to perform an altruistic act in a different capacity at some point in the future.[28] Following their extensive interviews with living donors, Bramstedt and Down found that 36 percent of living donors who gave their kidneys to strangers did so after becoming aware of another who had done the same, even if that knowledge came only from reading a book or watching a television show.[29] The psychologist Jonathan Haidt, who calls this phenomenon "elevation," quotes Thomas Jefferson to explain it:

Every thing is useful which contributes to fix us in the principles and practice of virtue. When any . . . act of charity or of gratitude, for instance,
is presented either to our sight or imagination, we are deeply impressed
with its beauty and feel a strong desire in ourselves of doing charitable and
grateful acts also. On the contrary when we see or read of any atrocious
deed, we are disgusted with its deformity and conceive an abhorrence of
vice. Now every emotion of this kind is an exercise of our virtuous dispositions; and dispositions of the mind, like limbs of the body, acquire strength
by exercise.[30]

Jefferson identifies one of the most profoundly impactful emotions in human
experience: our habit of being pre-reflectively inspired by moving examples of
loving acts of selfless behavior. Elevation is the emotion that creates "disciples
of goodness" by virtue of which paying it forward becomes a self-generating
occurrence.[31] At Haidt's urging this phenomenon has been empirically studied on many occasions, and multiple experiments now confirm that actors are
more likely to engage in altruistic behavior following their own observance of
instances of altruism.[32]

Returning to an earlier discussion, for the sake of argument let's suppose
that, relative to each other, being paid for donating an organ versus donating
one voluntarily without financial compensation produces the same level of
bad and good short- and long-term consequences. In other words, in terms
of the donor's well-being, we assume that being paid versus not being paid
is a wash. In this case, the findings of Bramstedt and Down, affirmed by
Haidt's research, still provide further reason for supporting a policy of not
paying donors: the phenomenon of elevation, in which wonderful behavior
is observed and then repeated by onlookers, is not triggered when the altru-
ist is being financially rewarded for his or her giving acts. Rather, the elevation occurs by a different mechanism altogether. This conclusion has support
from independent studies showing regional variation in living donor rates: in
regions with abounding examples of prosocial behavior of the sort shown to
increase subjective well-being, such as volunteering and charitable giving, the
prevalence of extraordinary acts of altruism, such as becoming a living donor,
also abound.[33] Environments that take on a communal character rather than
ones of isolated relationships governed by financial contractualism serve well-
being, which in turn further serves the performance of acts of extraordinary
altruism. We may conclude that the phenomenon of "elevation" should be
regarded as another reason among the preponderance of existing ones to favor

a system of organ procurement that does not rely on financial incentives to recruit living donors. That living donors come to be within the larger context of featured examples of prosocial behavior is a game changer.

REFLECTIONS OF A LIVING DONOR ADVOCATE

I live in New York, a state in which 27 percent of the residents are registered organ donors, as compared to a rate of close to 50 percent across the rest of the United States. This ranks New York last in the nation in the percentage of residents who are registered organ donors. While this figure applies to cadaveric donation—a designation most commonly noted by the presence of a heart on a driver's license—it also says something about the culture and arguably the legislative bureaucracy of the state. At a conference held at Stony Brook University in 2015 themed around the question of why New York has such low rates, one of the speakers made the point that there is so much paperwork associated with becoming an organ donor here, relative to other places, that many individuals never get the chance to explore the possibility of registering as an organ donor, a possibility that might well have been realized were people forced to jump through fewer hoops. This led me to wonder about the many areas of life in which, through no fault of our own, we are not given a natural occasion to reflect about what it would be like to become a living donor. We are in general not aware of the extent to which helping and caregiving behaviors fulfill human health and flourishing. Considering the work of health psychologists like Brown and Brown and others who have suggested a link between helping behaviors and happy living, one wonders if becoming a living donors would, in turn, make one a better friend, parent, or spouse, just as living donors sometimes report post-nephrectomy.[34] But recall the reason Amy Friedman offered for her reticence about becoming an unpaid living donor for a stranger: she is a mother, and such a decision could never sit well with her, as one day one of her own kids could need one of her kidneys.

There are now grounds to come to the opposite conclusion: donating an organ arguably makes one a better parent. This counterintuitive wisdom brings to mind a conversation I recently had with Dave Chameides, a dear friend of mine. In the 1990s Dave rode a bicycle across the United States, and then later down the West Coast, to raise awareness of HIV and AIDS. Ten years later Dave decided to keep all of the trash he and his family had accumulated for a full year (sorting his trash carefully and using worms to consume a lot of it in a contraption of his own making) in order to raise awareness about waste and the environment.[35] On the heels of these demanding, consciousness-raising activities he began to ask me questions about what steps he could take if he were interested in becoming a living donor.[36] When I shared with him the view of Amy Friedman and others whose cautions I respect—that as a parent he should think long and hard about this choice—he replied: "It is because I am a parent that I am seriously considering this. I am at my best as a parent when I am at my best for everyone, and besides, it is the example I want to set for my kids."

Dave's defense of his lifelong commitment to making the well-being of strangers a priority is noteworthy because it implies that such an ambition is of a piece rather than in competition with his obligations to his family. Often the principal objects of other-regard, between the near and dear and the impersonal stranger, stand in tension.[37] Dave, like some of the psychologists studying the health benefits of helping behaviors, sees things differently. His perception mirrors the sentiments I have often heard expressed since becoming a living donor advocate: subjects report, post-nephrectomy, that they have become better siblings, parents, children, friends, and people.

As a living donor advocate my "face time" with living donors takes place mostly prior to the surgery. However, by law living donor advocates must also meet with donors as they are recovering in the hospital twenty-four to forty-eight hours after surgery, just to check up on them and make sure they are satisfied (and attend to their concerns if they are not). These conversations are documented on their medical charts. Looking at my notes from these conversations over the past two years, some worthwhile impressions stick out (expressed in the words of donors themselves):

"I feel like a great weight has been lifted. I was so stressed before, and that stress is gone."

"This is the most important thing I have ever done in my life. I need to tell others to do it."

"I've never felt more human."

The most memorable was told to me by a woman who had just donated for her brother:

"I know in my heart that this experience has somehow made me a better mother."

My general sense in talking with many living donors is that, whether the recipient was a blood relative or not, the donors felt that donating a kidney was one of the most self-actualizing, confidence-building, and rewarding thing they had ever done, and something that freed them up afterward to be more available to others rather than holding them back. Becoming a donor had *given* them resources, not taken them away. In some cases these insights occurred after the fact. Many living donors don't fully consider what helping others might feel like or cause to change in them personally. Not to reflect too sentimentally or romantically on the process, there are certainly many occasions when the donor is simply exhausted, disoriented from pain medicine, or lacking the energy to say much of anything beyond that he or she is recovering and not in too much discomfort. Some of them, admittedly, have donated out of a feeling of duty and are not inclined to think too deeply beyond the idea that donating was something they felt they simply had to do. Even so, and despite the study in which 28 percent of living donors reported "feeling abandoned" in the days after surgery, I have yet to encounter such an individual myself. Everyone whose nephrectomy ended up taking place as planned reported a good experience with Stony Brook Hospital and expressed personal satisfaction with their decisions.

I have learned something else from donors. Prior to surgery, living donors tend to express a calm confidence about their plans. I rarely have witnessed fear, ambivalence, or the sort of stoic resignation that customarily comes with a decision that hasn't been so easy to make. This suggests to me that the commitment to donate an organ is not arrived at in a rationalistic manner, as would a life choice in which the brain, but not necessarily the heart, was on board. On the contrary, living donors have an inner yearning for what they are about to do. They don't *need* to donate to give their lives meaning—they are not like Dickens's Sydney Carton from *A Tale of Two Cities*, who redeemed himself in dramatic fashion in the final hour by trading in his own slovenly existence for a worthy better one, performing that "far, far better thing that I do, than I have ever done."[38] The act of the living donor is not desperate, nor rushed, nor foolhardy. It is, simply, something that makes sense in context, and part of an arc of the narrative one is in the process of creating about and for oneself. For just this reason it is sometimes difficult for me to recommend suspension of the process on the rare occasion when I believe it is inappropriate for a particular living donor to go through with his or her planned donation. This is because it is not merely a recipient who will have to wait longer to receive an organ; a donor's meaningful plans for himself or herself will also become frustrated. Living donor advocates must be careful to protect living donors physically but also in preserving their ability to self-determine. I have learned to harbor a healthy appreciation for donor autonomy, which is perhaps not so surprising given that my role as a living donor advocate is at times paternalistic. While I am present for donors' protection, and for the protection of all living donors in the transplantation process, there is at the same time a sense in which they know better than I ever could what they are about to do and why they are doing it.

These anecdotal and interview-based reflections confirm two claims about the nature of the relationship between altruism and self-regard on which evolutionary biologists, psychologists, philosophers, and theologians have increasingly come to concur: first, that self-regard and other-regard are not diametrical opposites but rather are the mutual fulfillment of one another; and second, that altruism, even in its most demanding expression, is not a saintly nor an exceptional activity that lies on the fringes of the best humanity has to offer. Rather, altruism is a positive, nurturing activity within the bell curve of normal human experience.[39]

Many evolutionary biologists have recently argued that we have evolved into organisms for whom our survival as a species has relied on our behaving in selfless ways for the sake of the perpetuation of our genes.[40] While these sacrifices mostly take the form of kin selection and reciprocal altruism, in terms of evolutionary advantage these selfless behaviors induce us to experience natural feelings of fulfillment.[41] In other words, to *be* a human individual organism that behaves the way it is supposed to behave (again, from a "gene's-eye-view") does not in all cases make its own individual survival paramount. By implication, authentic other-regard—of the kind that is not exclusively instrumental in service of self-regard—paradoxically becomes a primary interest of the self. This insight about biology is backed up by psychological mechanisms that human beings have developed over time to pattern their governing attitudes and motivations after this evolutionarily successful strategy. Already disposed to be altruistic in light of our biological makeup, we internalize other-regarding impulses, the overall effect of which is to further refine the instincts for sympathy and compassion that nature has provided us.

If other-regard and self-regard are coterminous in the process of human flourishing, then it follows that receiving is not the only component of altruistic giving wherein the participant benefits. To be altruistic is not just to bear the burden of costly giving. It is also to fulfill a need to give. Aside from the accumulating evidence to suggest that there are health advantages to living altruistically, at a prereflective level we are naturally sympathetic beings. Indeed, as early as eighteen months of age toddlers exhibit a desire to cooperate with those whom they perceive to have suffered in some way. In one significant series of experiments, psychologist Felix Warneken of the Max Planck Institute of Evolutionary Anthropology conducted a number of "tasks" in front of twenty-four eighteen-month-olds, such as piling up books and hanging towels up to dry, at times deliberately struggling with the tasks in order to see if that would elicit a response from the toddlers.[42] With remarkable consistency the toddlers would gesture to offer assistance on those occasions when Warneken framed the problem as one of needing help. (The toddlers withheld their assistance when Warneken intentionally took a book from the stack or let a towel fall by throwing a clothespin to the floor, implying that there was no one struggling or in need of assistance.) According to Warneken, in addition to having the cognitive ability to grasp people's goals and intentions at an early age, our "prosocial motivation" spurs us to feel connected to others by helping them when help appears needed.

In this sense we are beings whose happiness depends on making others happy. Were we to inhabit a different world, one in which no one suffered, we would be impoverished indeed. It would be myopic and perhaps a little offensive to contend that we are for this reason *better off* in a world that contains suffering than one bereft of it, particularly given the fact that the actual world in which we live contains such drastic and cruel instances of misery. While acknowledging this to be true, however, it is at the same time hard not to reflect on a silver lining: the suffering of others can bring out our better angels by reminding us of the humanity that connects us all to one another. In most cases, but for a stroke of luck the recipient could have been the donor, and vice versa. Moreover, in terms of how they see *themselves*, organ donors are no different than blood donors. Despite the major ordeal of surgery, they understand that they are doing something wonderful but not spectacular in the simultaneous service of humanity and their own personal growth and development. If we are really going to trust living organ donors not merely as the moral exemplars on whom we are ready to bestow praise but also as moral authorities who perhaps see something about the human experience that we do not yet see, then we should additionally take seriously their own sense that becoming a living donor isn't so crazy. It is, rather, a normal and healthy expression of human fulfillment.

To be fair, we have not yet arrived at that point in nephrectomy technology where giving one's kidney is as safe, easy, financially without burden, and free from potential long-term health consequences as is donating blood. Disincentives to becoming a living donor still abound, and their mitigation, if not removal, might go a long way toward inspiring more potential living donors to avail themselves of an activity that is part of normal human experience. Thus, we might need to attend to the more practical aspects of self-regard by removing disincentives in order to make more accessible the other, grander altruistic aspects of self-regard. What some of these measures might entail, and how to encourage selfless behaviors while not at the same time enabling exploitation, is the next subject for discussion.

NOTES

1. Immanuel Kant, *Groundwork of the Metaphysics of Morals*, trans. H. J. Paton (New York: Harper and Row, 1964), 67. Kant defined "moral duty" in this manner: we know for sure that we have done what we morally "ought" to have done only when we remove every possible reason, save for reverence for the moral law, for following a specific course of action. The moral law, in turn, is defined by the "categorical imperative," a procedural test according to which we should always act according to that maxim that we, at the same time, will to become a universal law. In other words, we ought not to make of our own case an exception or allow self-interest to have any direct or indirect say in morally directing us.

2. C. Daniel Batson and Laura L. Shaw, "Evidence for Altruism: Toward a Pluralism of Prosocial Motives," *Psychological Inquiry* 2, no. 2 (1991): 107–22.

3. C. Daniel Batson, *The Altruism Question: Toward a Social-Psychological Answer* (Hillsdale, NJ: Lawrence Erlbaum, 1991).

4. For a concrete example of this accusation in the case of one living donor, recall the case of Zell Kravinski. See Ian Parker, "The Gift," *New Yorker*, August 2, 2004, http://web.archive.org/web/20130912032748/http://www.stafforini.com:80/blog/the-gift/.

5. Jean Hampton, "Selflessness and the Loss of Self," in *Altruism*, ed. Ellen Frankel Paul, Fred D. Miller Jr., and Jeffrey Paul (Cambridge: Cambridge University Press, 1993), 135–65.

6. Aristotle, *Nicomachean Ethics*, trans. Terence Irwin (Indianapolis, IN: Hackett, 1985), 1169.

7. S. L. Brown, D. M. Smith, R. Schulz, M. U. Kabeto, P. A. Ubel, M. Poulin, and K. M. Langa, "Caregiving Behavior Is Associated with Decreased Mortality Risk," *Psychological Science* 20 (2009): 488–94; Stephen G. Post, ed., *Altruism and Health: Perspectives from Empirical Research* (Oxford: Oxford University Press, 2007).

8. While I have gotten permission from all three of these living donors to tell their stories, I have had contact with them only, and not their intended recipients, about whom much can also be inferred from these reports. Out of ample caution I have changed the names of both the donors and recipients.

9. This is precisely the concern with regard to Zell Kravinski, who has been accused of acting according to this sort of dispassionate utilitarian reasoning. See Parker, "The Gift."

10. Katrina A. Bramstedt and Rena Down, *The Organ Donor Experience: Good Samaritans and the Meaning of Altruism* (Lanham, MD: Rowman and Littlefield, 2011), 18.

11. Ibid., 19.

12. Ibid.

13. For a comprehensive defense of the position that the affective and cognitive components of emotions are in fact instances of one another—that is, that the emotions are, properly conceived, "judgments of value" not to be dismissed as irrational—see Martha Nussbaum, *Upheavals of Thought: The Intelligence of Emotions* (Cambridge: Cambridge University Press, 2001), esp. 19–88.

14. Bramstedt and Down, *Organ Donor Experience*, 20.

15. Ibid.

16. Ibid., 146.

17. Ibid., 150.

18. As reported by the United Network for Organ Sharing, last accessed August 16, 2016. See its website: https://www.unos.org/donation/living-donation/.

19. Highly sensitized patients and donors who have zero mismatches take precedence over prior living donors. I thank one of the anonymous reviewers for Georgetown University Press for pointing out these two exceptions.

20. P. M. Franklin and A. K. Crombie, "Live Related Renal Transplantation: Psychological, Social, and Cultural Issues," *Transplantation* 76 (2003): 1247–52.

21. E. M. Johnson et al., "Long-Term Follow-Up of Living Kidney Donors: Quality of Life after Donation," *Transplantation* 67 (1999): 717–21.

22. Bramstedt and Down, *Organ Donor Experience*, 153.

23. Ibid.

24. See Thomas Baumgartner et al., "Oxytocin Shapes the Neural Circuitry of Trust and Trust Adaptation in Humans," *Neuron* 58, no. 4 (2008): 639–50; and Stephanie L. Brown et al., "Social Closeness Increases Salivary Progesterone in Humans," *Hormones and Behavior* 56, no. 1 (2009): 108–11.

25. Stephanie L. Brown and Michael R. Brown, "Connecting Prosocial Behavior to Improved Physical Health: Contributions from the Neurobiology of Parenting," *Neuroscience and Biobehavioral Reviews* 55 (2015): 1–17.

26. Allan Luks and Peggy Payne, *The Healing Power of Doing Good* (Lincoln, NE: iUniverse, 2001), 10.

27. Margareta A. Sanner, "The Donation Process of Living Kidney Donors," *Nephrology Dialysis Transplantation* 20 (2005): 1707–13.

28. Bramstedt and Down, *Organ Donor Experience*, 161.

29. Ibid., 161–62.

30. Thomas Jefferson, "Letter to Robert Skipwith," in *The Portable Thomas Jefferson*, ed. M. D. Peterson (New York: Penguin, 1975), 349–51, quoted by Jonathan Haidt, "Disgust and Elevation: Opposing Sources of 'Spiritual Information,'" in *"Spiritual Information": One Hundred Perspectives*, ed. C. L. Harper Jr. (Philadelphia: Templeton Foundation, 2005), 426. Available at: http://www.happinesshypothesis .com/haidt.spiritual-information.pdf.

31. Haidt, "Disgust and Elevation," 427.

32. See Jonathan Haidt, "Elevation and the Positive Psychology of Morality," in *Flourishing: Positive Psychology and the Life Well-Lived*, ed. Corey L. M. Keyes and Jonathan Haidt (American Psychological Association, 2003), 275–89; Simone Schnall, Jean Roper, and Daniel Fessler, "Elevation Leads to Altruistic Behavior," *Psychological Science* 21, no. 3 (2010): 315–20; and Keith Cox, "Elevation Predicts Domain-Specific Volunteerism Three Months Later," *Journal of Positive Psychology* 5, no. 5 (2010): 333–41.

33. Kristin M. Brethel-Haurwitz and Abigail A. Marsh, "Geographical Differences in Subjective Well-Being Predict Extraordinary Altruism," *Psychological Science* 25, no. 3 (March 2014): 762–71.

34. Becoming a donor can also disrupt family relations. See Bramstedt and Down, *Organ Donor Experience*, 118–19.

35. For Dave's blog of his year keeping the entirety of his and his family's garbage in his basement, see Sustainable Dave's blog, *365 Days of Trash*, at http://365daysof trash.blogspot.com/.

36. I directed Dave to the UNOS link also provided above: https://www.unos .org/donation/living-donation/. Both websites last accessed August 16, 2016.

37. On the tension between the near and dear and the stranger as competing objects of other regard, see Andrew Michael Flescher and Daniel L. Worthen, *The Altruistic Species: Scientific, Philosophical, and Religious Perspectives of Human Benevolence* (Philadelphia: Templeton Foundation, 2007), 37. Two noteworthy examples of historical saintly souls renowned for their enormous efforts on behalf of humanity but who were less than ideal as husbands or fathers are Gandhi and Martin Luther King Jr. On Gandhi's success as a husband, see Jad Adams, *Gandhi: Naked Ambition* (London: Quercus, 2011). On Martin Luther King Jr.'s womanizing, see Michael Eric Dyson, *I May Not Get There with You: The True Martin Luther King, Jr.* (New York: Free Press, 2000), 216–22.

38. Charles Dickens, *Works of Charles Dickens: A Tale of Two Cities and Sketches by Boz* (New York: Kelmscott Society, 1904), 400.

39. Flescher and Worthen, *Altruistic Species*, 240–47.

40. Of the many sources appropriate for this citation remains Richard Dawkins, *The Selfish Gene*, 2nd ed. (Oxford: Oxford University Press, 1989).

41. Ibid.: on kin selection, see 88–107; on reciprocal altruism, see 183–88.

42. F. Warneken, F. Chen, and M. Tomasello, "Altruistic Helping in Human Infants and Young Chimpanzees," *Science* 311 (March 3, 2006): 1301–3.

5

Making Altruism Practical

To point out that we flourish when we sacrifice for others is not to say that sacrificing comes easily. As most clinicians and ethicists who work for the cause of organ transplantation are starting to realize, at present too many disincentives to donating exist, without which more people might become mobilized to consider living donation. There is a difference between adding a financial incentive and removing financial and other disincentives. In the first case the presumption is that incentives come primarily, if not exclusively, from financial reward; in the second, incentives remain intrinsic, but their appeal can seem distant or inaccessible so long as present hardships that emerge from the practical reality of taking steps to become a donor stand in the way of the larger altruistic ambition.

Some examples that remove disincentives to becoming an organ donor in service of making altruism "practical" include paired exchanges and larger "donor chains"; laws that give individuals preference when they opt into an organ donor network; financial assistance, direct or in the form of tax breaks, that provide compensation for travel or lost wages accrued in the donation process; additional benefits to donors or their families such as supplements to health insurance coverage; and sacred spaces, such as a "wall of heroes," which celebrate donors' willingness to sacrifice for others. All of these make the notion of "altruism" less fatuous and more doable. They represent practical ways of addressing or eliminating some of the real-world reasons people do not become living donors.

Knowing that civic duty is best fulfilled when we see ourselves as people tied together in a cohesive, communal collective rather than as individuals out for ourselves, nevertheless it should not be taken for granted that we will be receptive to forming bonds with others when we pay a price, individually, for trying to do so. As discussed earlier, the relative merits of introducing money into a system of the exchange of especially precious goods can, counterintuitively, turn out to be inefficient. Additionally, if folks sense that they stand to be exploited or neglected as they prepare to invest in others, they quickly become suspicious. Thus the signatories of the 2015 letter to Secretary of Health and Human Services Sylvia Mathews Burwell offer the following reality check:

> One major reason for the [organ shortage gap] is that living donors in the United States incur on average more than U.S. $6,000 in out-of-pocket costs. Potential donors may not be able to afford these expenses and may either be unaware of, or not meet the strict requirements for, programs that cover some but not all of donors' financial costs and losses.[1]

Not only are potential living donors not aware of the partial reimbursements they stand to receive for volunteering their organs; they must jump through hoops to make the case that they qualify for them.

On a legislative and bureaucratic level, we clearly do not make it easy for living donors to become their better selves, which indeed compromises the implicit campaign to earn the trust of potential donors on which a robust transplantation program would depend. As the few hundred signatories to the letter maintain, if we want to increase organ donation rates in the United States we must remove these financial disincentives. Being an organ donor should be a financially neutral act that "neither enriches living donors or the families of deceased donors nor burdens them with costs they would otherwise not face."[2]

The signers also aim to be comprehensive and fair in the reforms they suggest. For example, they note that while it is both more just and less expensive to prioritize transplantation over perpetual dialysis, in order to make the former a more realistic possibility we must alter our assumptions about the circumstances under which immunosuppressant drugs are provided for recipients, the cost of which currently is reimbursed for only three years. They enjoin us to rethink the living donation process altogether through the creation of a task force to come up with new ideas consistent with the spirit of the National Transplantation Act of 1984, which prohibits giving "valuable consideration" in exchange for an organ.

How far we can legitimately stretch the interpretation of the prohibition against valuable consideration is the subject of much debate. Does the prohibition apply strictly to financial reward, for example, or does it also proscribe even-exchange trade of comparably precious commodities such as education, retirement benefits, health or other forms of insurance, or even partial or full mortgage forgiveness? While we might guess what Kant would say, the differences between the variously proposed exchanges, as well as the differences between the various goods just mentioned and the value of lump-sum monetary payment, matter. Do they or don't they represent an in-principle violation of the prohibition against receiving remuneration for an organ? How can we implement best practices with regard to living donation programs across the country that optimize education, access, and care, while doing so in an ethically sound manner? We will first consider ideas that don't have indirect monetary implications and then address the compatibility of exchanging highly valuable "non-liquid" goods with the regulations currently in effect.

PAIRED EXCHANGES AND DONOR CHAINS

There is arguably no incentive stronger than the desire to satisfy the desperate needs of a loved one. Unfortunately, not every family member is in a position to do so, even when it is a sibling, child, or cousin in need. In fact, the majority of family members are not compatible.[3] When a match cannot be found within the family, the hopeful recipient must find another suitable match. This process, as the example of Sally Satel shows (see chap. 1), is extremely stressful for the one pressed with the burden of finding an unrelated but willing suitable donor. Thankfully, technology, and in particular our refined ability to locate matched strangers through sophisticated mathematical models, has made this somewhat less tragic.

Models can now help locate strangers who may not be a match for a loved one but who, at the same time, have a loved one for whom they themselves are not a match but *are* suitable for the very individual in the same situation. In these paired exchanges—when there are two pairs of individuals incompatible with each other but who are, in both cases, compatible with the other's loved one—donors and recipients of both pairs "swap," making two transplantations possible. In a manner that could have hardly been envisioned on a practical level prior to the advent of the Internet, with timeliness and confidence donors and recipients, even those living in different parts of the country, can be matched. The Organ Procurement and Transplantation Network

(OPTN) managed by the United Network for Organ Sharing (UNOS) now exists precisely to facilitate such introductions, which hopefully result in good outcomes for everyone involved. The main promise of a paired exchange, ethically and otherwise, is that a precious good (a bodily organ) is being volunteered by a willing donor for a return of the *exact same* especially precious good: there is no apparent conflict of interest, no cause to worry about coercion, no need for money to facilitate the crucial exchange. Technology itself has beautifully and parsimoniously made all of this possible.

The OPTN makes paired exchanges accessible and affordable for the public by contracting through the Health Resources and Services Administration (HRSA), the agency of the US Department of Health and Human Services (DHS) under whose purview the regulation of transplantations in our country falls. The OPTN registers and carefully monitors everyone who signs up for the program, which becomes a database that allows transplant centers and organ recovery agencies throughout the United States to optimize the matching of initially incompatible donor pairs with suitable alternative pairs.[4] Joining the program is relatively easy: a prospective recipient must merely be receiving care at a transplant center in the United States, even if this care is being rendered prior to the recipient going on dialysis. There is no cost to join. Neither recipients nor donors are involved in the payment or receipt of money at registration. And in most (but not all) cases, the matched recipient's health insurance pays for any costs associated with the medical evaluation of the donor prior to surgery.[5] Matching occurs by way of assigned transplant coordinators availing themselves of the computerized system to see which registrants are willing to travel certain distances or, depending on the circumstances, willing to accept shipped kidneys.[6] Ideally, nephrectomies arranged as a result of paired exchanges take place on the same day.

Paired exchanges have not only revolutionized the manner in which individuals who lack a suitable family match can avoid the desperate search to find someone else; the nature of the exchange itself is such that it is purified of ethical complications, since there is no deliberation to figure out whether or not a donor's sacrifice is being met with appropriate compensation. Presumably in paired exchanges it is love that motivates both donors and gratitude that fills up both recipients. That technology facilitates the process is a grace. Its upshot is to relieve the pressures otherwise building up on a system already weighed down by shortage. Additionally, the presumption of trust on the part of all four individuals is the irreplaceable glue that upholds the practice of organ transplantation in the first place—not a bad thing on which to depend in the context of a paired exchange. We are today only beginning to see the promising advantages of the possibility of paired exchanges to living donor programs.[7]

When paired exchanges move beyond just four or six individuals, the multiple bodily organ swaps are called "chains." In February 2011 a donor chain involving sixty lives and thirty kidneys was put into motion when Rick Ruzzamenti, who runs a yoga studio in Riverside, California, heard his receptionist tell him she had recently donated a kidney to a friend in need whom she had bumped into at Target. The story so captured Ruzzamenti's attention that two days later he contacted Riverside Community Hospital to inquire into how he might go about doing the same thing.[8] Later that year, a desperate patient who'd received a dire diagnosis of diabetes-related renal disease while still in his mid-forties but who could not find a suitable donor among his immediate friends of family became the fortunate last individual among twenty-nine others to receive a new functioning kidney in a transplantation procedure that took place at Loyola University Medical Center in Chicago.[9] The story reported by Kevin Sack in the *New York Times* of how all sixty participants became linked, beginning with one altruistic donor and ending with one needy recipient, elucidates what makes donor chains such a promising way forward in the bid to make a real dent in the organ shortage gap:

> What made the domino chain of 60 operations possible was the willingness of a Good Samaritan, Mr. Ruzzamenti, to give the initial kidney, expecting nothing in return. Its momentum was then fueled by a mix of selflessness and self-interest among donors who gave a kidney to a stranger after learning they could not donate to a loved one because of incompatible blood types or antibodies. Their loved ones, in turn, were offered compatible kidneys as part of the exchange. Chain 124, as it was labeled by the nonprofit National Kidney Registry, required lockstep coordination over four months among 17 hospitals in 11 states.[10]

It should immediately strike anyone considering the innovation of donor chains that the nature of the bulk of its participants' motivation is a spirit of paying it forward, empowered by the acute self-interest one feels to help a loved one. Chains allow the possibility of indirectly giving to a loved one and doing so without, again to borrow Sandel's language, the "corrupting" effect of money. This is no small feat. But with sophisticated algorithms neither is it impossible to link sixty individuals as compatibly suitable in the precise manner they all can turn out to be, though perhaps it is even more remarkable that not one of the sixty people in the Ruzzamenti chain changed his or her mind.

One of the perils with chains, as with any planned paired exchange, or even transplantation occurring between just two individuals, is that at any moment any potential donor fully has the right to, and can, back out. Everyone has a personal life that entails mood swings, emergencies, and garden-variety fear. The promise to donate one's organ is precarious right up to the moment of the nephrectomy, whether two individuals, let alone sixty people, are depending on one another. By the same token, as Sack notes, a leap of faith taken by one person inspires subsequent ones.

The main risk with chains is that someone reneging remains a possibility until the last nephrectomy and transplantation have been performed. This noted, within five years of their inception and first attempt in 2005 at Johns Hopkins University, chains and other forms of paired exchange have resulted in nearly five hundred transplants being performed in this country per year. This is a figure that experts predict could increase eightfold if Americans became more aware about programs putting eligible donors and recipients in contact with one another.[11]

Chains in and of themselves are not the answer, but they are a piece of the overall puzzle: they capture both the "pay it forward" attitude by which organic motivation to help the neighbor is engendered and they appeal to the self-regard that viscerally grabs a giver's attention to a desperate recipient in need. Computer-generated algorithms help to make sure that geographical barriers are no longer an insurmountable issue for willing donors. Today, new biotechnical companies are sprouting up to enable transplantation centers all over the country to maximize efficiency in facilitating matches, which meets compliance regulations in a way that assures the highest-quality care to donors and recipients.[12] Notwithstanding the danger that chains can be broken, they do provide wonderful publicity to the cause of organ donation and power the "elevation" phenomenon described by Jonathan Haidt (see chap. 4). Through example, more willing donors are inspired to step forward. As technology advances and educational initiatives sprout across the country, no doubt chains will become a bigger part of the solution to closing the gap between those needing an organ and those with organs who are willing to donate.

CREATING INCENTIVES TO OPT IN

Unlike the situation in twenty-four countries in Europe, which presume that upon death one's organs will become available to be transplanted into the body of another if the organs are suitable, the United States has only an "opt-in" policy for cadaveric donation. The requirement to register proactively to become an organ donor is something that can happen ad hoc when obtaining a driver's license or stumbling across an organ donor drive but, depending on the state in which one resides, it also can be bureaucratically complicated. The rationale behind an opt-in over an opt-out system is that genuine informed consent requires making sure anyone who becomes an organ donor is explicitly made aware of what it entails. In theory this includes the opportunity for the prospective donor to familiarize himself or herself with the available literature, a time to discuss options with healthcare providers, and a time to consider the ramifications on work and family before making the decision about what to do with one's body parts after one dies. Unfortunately, and despite the best intentions of an opt-in rationale, many people never get the chance to make this informed decision as a result of resource-strapped motor vehicle departments, the arbitrary nature of the location and timing of organ donation registration drives, and the relatively low publicity accorded the cause of organ donation in the first place. It is indeed difficult to engender enthusiasm for organ donor registration drives in lieu of effective incentives, monetary or otherwise.

In response to unusually low donation rates, one country has pioneered a new system to increase organ donation rates by appealing to self-regard in an innovative manner. Prior to 2012, Israel ranked at the bottom in terms of participating donor registrants, even among all opt-in Western countries. This was largely due to three reasons: (1) the widespread view that the dead ought not to be desecrated, despite the custom in the Jewish tradition that "necessity overrides prohibition" and that organ donation is not just an allowable practice but a virtuous one; (2) issues surrounding the legitimacy of brain death; and (3) the fact that observant Haredi Jews, while free to accept organs from other donors should the need arise, are not allowed to become donors themselves, according to most rabbis in their communities.[13] In response, Israel decided to experiment with a new policy giving transplantation priority to patients who have previously agreed to donate their organs, thereby making the country the first in the world to make non-need-related (i.e., nonmedical) criteria relevant to one's position on the waiting list.[14]

Reflecting on the unfairness of a system that failed to reward those who buy into it, Dr. Jacob Lavee, a cardiothoracic surgeon in charge of the heart transplantation program of Sheba Medical Center in Tel Hashomer, spearheaded the new proposal. With the help of rabbis, lawyers, physicians, and medical ethicists, he worked to enact a new law, unprecedented worldwide, that (all other things being equal) put those in need of a new organ to the top of the list if they had indicated a willingness to donate as well.[15] The passage of the new law

> was accompanied by a huge public awareness campaign about organ donation, with radio, TV, billboard and newspaper ads promoting the new priority system and countering the perception that Jewish law forbids donation. Shopping centers and coffee houses were blanketed with organ donation information. The response was overwhelming, as people registered in droves as potential donors.
>
> "We were swamped," says Tamar Ashkenazi, the director of the National Transplant Center of Israel. The machine that prints the organ donation cards usually handles 3,000 a month—5,000 if two workers are dedicated full-time to operating it. During the 10 weeks of the publicity campaign, 70,000 Israelis registered for organ donation cards. The consent rate from families . . . increased, and the number of organs available for patients has increased in parallel. Transplants . . . increased by more than 60 percent over all this year.[16]

The proposal worked, in a manner that did not bring money into the conversation. Initially nicknamed "Don't Give, Don't Get" because of the explicit tie between a self-regarding pay-off and an essentially other-regarding act, the new law met with controversy; for instance, the system gives advantage only to those candidates in the same tier of need and does not sanction the catapulting of less-needy candidates over more-needy ones. It remains unclear how much of a difference the law will ultimately make in organ donation. But even so, within just one year of its inception Israeli participation rates jumped dramatically higher from the level they were the year before.[17]

The Israeli law involves cadaveric donation, but I bring it up because it represents yet another example of thinking outside the box in order to align selfless and self-regarding motives without resorting to financial incentives. Following the Israeli experiment, other countries, such as the United Kingdom, began to consider following suit.[18] Such policies presume an attitude of

"We are all in this together." Though not coercive, they do put the plight of one's fellow citizens front and center: but for the grace of God it could be you who finds yourself in desperate need tomorrow, so today it behooves you to think about those who suffer and are waiting. Self-interest has helped kick-start virtue until the time when virtue alone is the primary driver.

LOST WAGES AND TRAVEL EXPENSES

Returning to the case of living donation, the explicit issue of costs borne by living donors in the process of making their altruistic gesture must be considered. More than any other factor, financial hardship motivated the 2015 letter to the head of DHS, urging her to set in motion legislation that would encourage living donor participation by making it a "financially neutral act."[19] All living donors must take two to three weeks off from work, even if their jobs do not entail much in the way of physical activity. Additionally, after the 24–48 hours spent in the hospital, they should spend at least ten more days before traveling (usually back home). And someone will need to assist them for the duration. All of these cost time and money and disrupt the life of anyone who is not independently wealthy or who will not face consequences from taking off significant time from work. The signatories to the letter to DHS sensibly proposed that Medicare or other comparable insuring agents should cover all of the "inconvenience" costs donors bear in putting themselves forward, not just because donors should be thanked rather than burdened for their sacrifice, nor only because we should not have a policy that makes only the rich and comfortable able to avail themselves of it. Rather, it is because compensating donors makes economical sense too.

As a society we have already decided to pay for dialysis. The expenditures for patients with end-stage renal disease add up. Beyond year one, it is significantly more expensive to treat patients on dialysis than it is to treat those who have received a donated kidney. Providing help to potential donors to address the many financial burdens they face upon donating is an investment in the transition from treatment of end-stage renal disease via dialysis to treatment through transplantation.

Compensating living donors for the financial hardships is an idea that already has gained limited traction. In the United States, the National Living Donor Assistance Center (NLDAC) offers financial support to facilitate the travel of living donors when the recipient's insurance company refuses coverage. Donors can receive a credit card to cover all eligible expenses, including transportation, food, lodging, and travel for the donor's support person, up to $6,000.[20] To qualify for this assistance both the donor and recipient must be US citizens (or lawfully admitted residents) and the *recipient's* household income (not the donor's) must be less than 300 percent of the federal poverty guidelines.[21] While the donor's household income informs the determination, it is the recipient who must request financial assistance on behalf of the donor. This is significant, for it underscores the degree to which the situations of the recipient and donor are linked, besides in the obvious medical sense.

While it is usually the living donor coordinator's job to apply for this financial assistance on behalf of the recipient-donor pair, should the money for some reason fail to come through, NOTA *does* allow for the recipient to provide financial assistance to the donor directly so long as this assistance is deemed within the margin of "reasonable payments" customarily associated with the expenses of travel, housing, and lost wages. Again, this is worth noting. Despite the fact that our legal system arguably doesn't go far enough in terms of reaching the goal of financial neutrality, it does make a distinction between what constitutes "reasonable compensatory payment" and "lump-sum financial reward," which presumably mirrors the difference between safeguarding against exploitation and offering enticements through means of a thoroughgoing self-interested incentive. In the former case the altruistic impulse is left intact, while in the latter it is undermined. The adjustment needed to improve the system is therefore not qualitative. We already have a precedent in place for compensating donors whose gesture places them under duress. At this point we need merely to make it easier for donors to receive compensation, clarify who will be the payers, and perhaps increase the amount they are compensated.

This becomes a particularly important thing to do in light of the reality that a recipient's financial standing bears a great deal on his or her ability to quickly travel through the waiting line, appear on multiple waiting lists, and ultimately receive an organ.[22] Since the wealthier one is, the more likely it will be that he or she knows other individuals of means, improvements to the criteria for eligibility for financial assistance (as well as better processing itself, facilitated through NLDAC) become even more important. To be sure, improvements are likely to make a big impact on both increasing the available pool of organs and on making organs more accessible to underprivileged populations. At the moment, wealthier people are in a more advantageous position to afford the needed tests and travel to meet potential recipients; UNOS does not presently ban or even limit multiple listings.[23] Dr. Raymond Givens, lead author of a study that examined the Scientific Registry of Transplant Recipients database, has demonstrated a link between wealth and successful matches through to transplantation. Givens worries that the advantage to those with means is an affront to the principle of transplanting the sickest and neediest patients first, and certainly of not discriminating against them if they lack resources.[24]

If we desire to remove participation impediments to most people, in particular impediments for those financially struggling, then we must do a better job of eliminating the barriers that rightly give this majority pause when they consider stepping up to the plate for another.[25] And, to repeat, to address the needs of this relatively impoverished demographic is to everyone's benefit in terms of preserving overall resources in the system. Indeed, for both moral and economic reasons, in the future we must do a better job of leveling the playing field so that the *only* issue a prospective living donor must consider is whether or not he or she has the courage and determination to engage in this admittedly onerous form of civic fellowship. The laws currently on the books need modification in order to make this decision the one that is front and center.

PUBLICLY ACKNOWLEDGING LIVING DONORS

Finding intelligent ways of incentivizing participation is not merely a matter of removing impediments; it entails making use of positive motivations as well. What can we do to appeal to the part of ourselves that naturally and appropriately lights up when we are acknowledged for the difference we make in the lives of others? Or, to put the matter more technically, how do we engender on a widespread basis Haidt's spirit of elevation, which, when it becomes manifest, also becomes self-perpetuating? To take a minor example, in Sweden when someone donates blood, the donor receives an SMS text message each time his or her specific volume of blood is used in the service of saving a life.[26] But that is not all. Over time the text messages continue to come, and the donor learns the long-term impact of his or her donation. This system serves not only as a richly deserved thanks but also as a reminder to the donor to donate more blood in the future and encourages, by word of mouth, others to do the same.

These kinds of innovation, which cost next to nothing and are easily amenable to amplification through social media, not surprisingly make reporting on and responding to the national blood donor registry in Sweden that much more efficient. On the official website of Stockholm's blood service a chart posts a running total of how much blood of each type and subtype is left in stock, how much is needed, and where civic response would make the most difference.[27] In a study conducted in 2013 at Johns Hopkins University, researchers found that social media multiplied the number of people who registered themselves as organ donors by twenty-one times the normal amount within a single day, giving direct evidence to the effectiveness of social norming in blood and organ donation campaigns.[28] According positive publicity to altruistic gestures has the potential to impact registration rates. Furthermore, such advertisement is not coercive, as are arguably massive propaganda campaigns among captive audiences in fútbol stadiums in Spain and elsewhere in Europe, where the government inundates its audience with messaging justifying its opt-out system of cadaveric donation. By contrast, fact-sensitive education exists in service of inspiring but not unduly forcing a better society than the one we currently inhabit.

One highly effective way of celebrating and educating our citizenry occurs when healthcare-providing institutions that facilitate organ transplantations feature recognition events that give organ donors the opportunity to share their personal stories with the public. By witnessing their courage, others can both admire and consider possibly emulating it one day. Donor celebration events clearly state that what might have seemed like a fatuous possibility is in fact a doable reality for most anyone.

The United Network for Organ Sharing honors organ and tissue donors at the National Donor Memorial, a ten-thousand-square-foot memorial garden located in Richmond, Virginia. Featured in the central room of the garden is the "wall of names" of donors who made the gift of life, as well as the words "Hope, Renewal, Transformation" engraved into a bronze medallion in the granite surface.[29] Every year a Donor Memorial Award for Excellence is bestowed on the "unsung heroes" who have gone above and beyond the call of duty in bringing awareness to the cause of organ donation in their communities. The National Donor Memorial includes a butterfly garden, a "wall of tears" to pay tribute to donors' families and their loved ones, and an interactive kiosk with Internet-based accounts of specific donor stories. The memorial as a whole celebrates the interconnectedness of all human life and the difference we always stand to make in the lives of others, even in the worst of times.

Many donor celebration events occur locally as well. For example, LiveOnNY has just opened an art installation in East Meadow, New York, named *The Grieving Wall*. Like the Western Wall in Jerusalem, the exhibit allows participants to express their feelings about lost loved ones (who in this case were also organ donors) on cards that are attachable to the wall in such a way that their messages can be easily accessed and read by others.[30] The artist, Panisa Khunprasert, hopes the installation not only facilitates coping with loss but also creates a communal environment in which grievers and recipients and their families can celebrate the sacrifice of donors together, even if not in the same moment. LiveOnNY now organizes walks to the destination of Khunprasert's *Grieving Wall* among donor families, transplant recipients, and others interested in the cause of organ donation. Such one-day events become, in the words of its brochure, "a road traveled together" at the end of which a thriving community of different constituents becomes ever broadened.

While "wall of heroes" events such as these national and local ones usually pertain to tragic instances of cadaveric donation (although often living donors are also honored), they are relevant to our topic of living donation insofar as they provide the opportunity for donor families to reinforce positively the noble good free of the inducement of money. One can consistently observe the degree to which family members of their beloved deceased are comforted by the notion that such great good is able to come from tragedy. Almost without exception a bond develops between the families of donors and recipients. They enjoy summer cookouts together, share friends and acquaintances in common, and eagerly mark their calendars in anticipation of honorary events celebrating the gift of life. Living donors maintain an active presence on these occasions, particularly in the case of individuals who have donated a kidney to someone who was not a family member. After attending many of these events, not once have I heard any individuals express a desire for monetary compensation in return for their sacrifice—but I have frequently witnessed them inspiring others listening in to their stories, investigating what it might take to walk down a similar path.

NONMONETARY VALUABLE, COMPARABLE GOODS

Some believe that while it is ethically problematic to pay living donors for their organs, we should nevertheless be doing more than the law currently allows to compensate tangibly those whose significant sacrifice of a bodily organ saves the life of another. They suggest going beyond the premise of paired exchanges to one based on "comparable goods." With comparable goods the exchange occurs under the presumption that the sacrificer receives a good of equal value, if not specifically a "reward," to make up for the hardship he or she endures in the sacrifice and despite the fact that a lump sum of money is deliberately left out of the equation. Examples of such comparable goods may be health insurance benefits for a period of time, a portion of college tuition, a substantial stipend toward a professional degree, or a "bankable" promise of credit, or a voucher, for some future need. Arguably comparable goods are somewhat similar to the goods of a collective character examined earlier, which Bruno Frey and his colleagues have proposed (see chap. 3). In contrast to lump-sum payments, these goods could compensate burdened citizens for sacrificing for their nation. Given that the compensation being received is not of an individual nature to be used exclusively at the receiver's discretion, a further argument can be made that comparable goods are communal and thus conducive to civic engagement insofar as they promote education and health in general. The promise of comparable goods certainly appeals to our self-interest, but it also lubricates the wheels of civic engagement.[31]

On the other hand, it is no secret that the examples just cited cost a good deal of money—that is, money that the donor will save in return for donating. Furthermore, it is not entirely clear that despite the fact that comparable goods implicitly refer to communal values (e.g., education), they retain their communal character given that they would be individually rendered. Real questions need to be asked about whether a proposed compensatory good serves a larger communal value. One instance where the idea of a "bankable credit" has decidedly cleared the burden of communal cooperation is occurring at UCLA in a new pilot program that is already showing early signs of success. The program, based on a voucher system, enables living donors to donate a kidney in advance of the time when they expect that a friend or family member might require a kidney transplant.[32]

A few things recommend this idea as a smart and ethically sound way of tapping into self-regarding motivation without also invoking the corrupting influence of money. First, it allows for unprecedented flexibility in the transplantation process. Maybe the donor is aging and wants his or her organ to be completely viable when it is removed, which it might not be by the time the proposed recipient needs it. In this case, "banking virtue" by keeping a record of what the donor has done allows the possibility that the donor's loved one will be a prioritized recipient later on, when the time is appropriate. This is essentially a paired exchange but one that is staggered over a period of months or years. As Dr. Jeffrey Veale, the transplant surgeon who helped implement the program at UCLA, explains, the arrangement is, not surprisingly, the idea of a grandfather named Howard Broadman, a lawyer and retired judge from Laguna Niguel, California, who was eager to donate a kidney to his grandson who was nearing but not quite yet at dialysis dependency. Broadman felt he would be too old to donate when his grandson finally needed him to do so. He is a good example of someone who, due to timing alone, would probably not have been a living donor were it not for the "bankable good" program that is able to guarantee that his virtuous sacrifice corresponds to the self-regarding pay-off on behalf of his grandson down the line.

A second advantage pertains to Haidt's observations about the phenomenon of elevation and the creation—via self-regard—of opportunities to be other-regarding. Here, virtue literally presents its own reward. The program Veale has implemented at UCLA organically allows organ donation to be given a wide hearing; the idea of residing on a waiting list is now something more than a particular determination at one snapshot in time. Veale's program is in this respect a cognate of the new policy in Israel, in which buy-in to the registry elevates one's place on the donor waiting list. In both instances an altruistic ambition is served by self-regard but in a way that gives greater publicity to the larger cause.

Unless one is a purist who believes that no self-interest can result from an altruistic act, this approach is free and clear of ethical qualms and a smart way of addressing the organ shortage crisis and fueling overall buy-in. Based on this reasoning, Veale hopes his program will induce more donors to step forward who, unlike Howard Broadman, have no particular future recipient's welfare in mind at the time they are poised to undergo a nephrectomy but who will leave the operation with a voucher in hand for a directed donation, should the occasion ever arise down the line when someone they know needs a kidney. Presumably, if enough people act according to this essentially altruistic but self-regardingly spiced logic, the bank of organs will grow and the waiting list will diminish.

Should vouchers be allowed to be issued not for the same good of a future transplanted kidney but for another comparable benefit? This question is trickier. First of all, it is not clear what might be equitably regarded as "comparable"; second, even if such a determination could be made, we should not take it for granted that such a good would be universally perceived as comparable. Doing so opens up the possibility that such exchanges of non-exact goods could be perceived as arbitrary or subjective assignments of value with respect to those who might be exploited in the proposed exchange. As even Robert Veatch, a proponent of the idea of selling organs, notes, any payment or receipt of a valuable good in exchange for an organ is apt to be "perceived differently by different people in different financial situations."[33] This reality, in which a kidney is not exchanged for a kidney, leads to a possible "slippery slope" of objections. For example, if we determine that donating a kidney confers the right to trade in a credit for premier health insurance coverage for a period of time, or indefinitely, then other questions emerge: Am I unduly advantaged because I am in a position to donate my kidney and someone else isn't? Should my ability to donate a kidney entitle me to comprehensive health insurance coverage? Something less? Something more? And what of the temptation to ask these sorts of questions? Will they lead me to become a kind of human calculator, where I pay close attention to what I have coming to me relative to what I've given up? In the long run, how conducive *is* an elaborate system that involves the exchange of comparable goods (in lieu of lump-sum payments) to creating the sort of communal culture we want? Finally, who are the legitimate authorities by which the relative value of comparable goods are fairly assessed? While it is relatively easy to make the case that a kidney is worth a kidney (overlooking the truism that no two kidneys are in exactly the same shape at the time they are removed from one body and transplanted into another), the case quickly gets complicated when we start to replace one sort of especially precious valuable good with another. Questions about exploitation do not lend themselves to consideration in the first scenario (of a kidney for a kidney) as easily as they do in the second (a kidney for a comparable good).

Whether the good in question is lifelong health insurance, tax credits, educational tuition vouchers, or contribution to tax-free retirement accounts, even when it is the government, and not individual recipients, that is compensating donors with these goods, problems immediately arise when calculations start being made about whether or not such goods are *really* commensurate with one another. In such calculations a psychology of counting surfaces and, in turn, monopolies of self-interest come to occupy the space of shared motivation.

While ideally self-sustaining, virtue itself, as well as a communal spirit, are delicate and dependent on widespread trust. As Martha Nussbaum has persuasively argued, both are "fragile" states conducive to human flourishing.[34] Introduce self-regarding motivation with too heavy a hand and the spirit of collaborative ambition will give way to the attitude of "everyone out for oneself." In addition to the possibility of creating this kind of negative chain of events, there is also a risk that the "pay it forward" spirit of giving becomes diluted. A system whereby kidneys are exchanged for kidneys, even in cases when the return gift is banked, plausibly remains consistent with the collaborative and communal spirit of widespread buy-in to the goal of pursuing public betterment. However, lifelong health insurance or tuition vouchers that can save hundreds of thousands of dollars in a few short years could be seen as massive compensatory rewards that are not all that different from financial payouts, making the preservation of this spirit not so certain. Thus, while such exchanges are not the same thing as receiving cash for organs, it is not all that easy to make the case that permitting them preserves the intention of the 1984 National Organ Transplantation Act, as proponents often argue.

This point noted, we might consider as a society experimenting with *measured* forms of compensation using comparable goods. As Veatch and others have proposed, living donors, for example, might be given some special consideration, what Veatch terms "bonus points," should they become ill in the future, whether or not becoming ill is a result of their prior nephrectomy.[35] One interesting idea has been put forward by Richard Schwindt and Aidan Vining. They suggest a "mutual insurance pool" in which an individual in the pool would receive priority for his or her organs from other members if he or she agreed to make organs available in the event of death.[36] Other minor incentives could be introduced to induce participation, such as invitations to events on specific days per year in which major theme parks like Disney World opened their doors to living donors, or catered mass benefits featuring major musical or comical acts, each with the purpose of honoring the donor who sacrificed his or her organ. No doubt the line beyond which a token gift becomes an unacceptable lure is murky, just as it is in other cases in medical ethics, but guidelines for such a line could reasonably be probed, as long as such gifts remained relatively minor. The larger point, as it has been in the case of the other sorts of incentives short of paying the donor that we have considered in this chapter, is one of availing ourselves of innovation for the sake of efficiency. Without making any major sacrifice along moral lines, we can, if we think creatively enough, do much to alter head-on the reality of the current national waiting list for organs.

HELPING VIRTUE ALONG

Should altruism need to be helped along? As the saying goes, virtue is its own reward. But sometimes on a practical level the idea of virtue might need a little push on behalf of the one destined to act virtuously. Civic duty, as a kind of experiment, is a counterintuitive alternative to the commonsensical proposition that financial reward is most likely to incentivize people to do something as costly or demanding as donating a bodily organ. It stands to reason that like many experiments, the "civic duty solution" may need activation energy to get it going. Giving virtue a little push, and certainly removing the disincentives to its performance, may go a long way. However, a balance must be struck between creating optimal conditions by which to give virtue a chance and not overwhelming virtue with powerful self-interested inducements. As noted earlier, offering large sums of money for the performance of self-sacrificial deeds has the psychological effect of making the gesture the only significant one. Once money is introduced, the definition of the transaction changes and comes to acquire a contractual nature.

Proponents and opponents of legalizing the sale of organs agree that our current system is inadequate; the waiting list has grown consistently over the last twenty years. Something has to change. Educating the public about living donations programs represents a key initiative to raising awareness about the plight of people on dialysis or in organ failure. But, as almost anyone working in organ transplantation would agree, this campaign would at least be enhanced—without any significant ethical cost—by implementing or further developing the proposals presented here. Unfortunately, our better angels are not always so quick to be released. While humans are not at base self-interested beings, nor are we purely altruistic beings ceaselessly devoted to promoting others in the abstract. Rather, we are relational, social beings; as such we are vulnerable and we harbor the need to connect with others. We display a preference for replenishing the needs of others as we fulfill needs of our own.

These proposals collectively have in common the feature of making it easier for us to be available for others. Paired exchanges and chains take into account the reality that not everyone is a suitable match for his or her loved one, and that matched strangers are often geographically remote from one another, and who, without technology, would otherwise have no means of coming into contact. Programs to compensate donors for lost wages or travel expenses incurred in the process of organ transplantation can ease the burdens or roadblocks by which one's impulse to help another might be thwarted because of the reality that often donors simply cannot afford it. While paired exchanges and chains as well as living donor assistant programs both have shown to be effective in removing some of the barriers to having more living donors step forward, much more could be done.

In the same respect, events acknowledging the contributions of donors—whether living or cadaveric—could occur more regularly, as currently happens with blood donation. When the good and worthwhile efforts of organizations like UNOS and Donate Life start to occur on a more frequent and regular basis, we can expect to see a positive impact on the waiting list. We don't know the long-term effectiveness of "banking" the sacrifice one makes in stepping forward to donate a bodily organ for another; but while it is largely untested and closer to the edge of the envelope than the other examples considered, it is, as experts point out, also promising. Currently, save for a few regions of the country, the law only allows for kidney or liver donors to go to near the top of the waiting list should the time come when they need a transplantation; there are no other nonmonetary benefits they can expect to receive down the line as a result of their sacrificial act.[37] Whether or not there should be at least warrants more thought and conversation.

In the end, whatever changes to NOTA we decide as a society to make, these changes should reflect the complementary ambitions of enhancing our motivation to share in the alleviation of the suffering of those in organ failure and of widening the "donate for life" community by inclusively bringing together its various constituents from the donor and the recipient side. Offering exclusively financial incentives for sacrifice pushes us toward individualism and the corresponding strategy of looking out for number one. The introduction of self-regarding but nonfinancial incentives seems to do the opposite. Like all experiments, the constructive proposals presented here could fail. But, especially given the advancing frontiers of technology, where we now have the medical means and clinical skill to make a difference in the lives of others like never before, it behooves us to try new things. Doing nothing, or even just passively leaving donor registration rates at the mercy of the wheels of bureaucracy, is no longer the most intelligent or compassionate option.

NOTES

1. "An Open Letter to President Barack Obama, Secretary of Health and Human Services Sylvia Mathews Burwell, Attorney General Eric Holder, and Leaders of Congress," September 11, 2014. See: http://ustransplantopenletter.org/openletter.html.

2. Ibid.

3. Among family members, it is most likely that a donor who is a sibling will be a suitable match for a recipient. Determining whether or not one is eligible to be a donor is a matter of testing for HLA, or Human Leukocyte Antigen. The HLA test examines genetic markers on white blood cells, where the immune system that helps protect the body against infectious disease and foreign invaders is located. If the recipient's markers are similar enough to the donor's, they may be a match. While siblings are the most likely to have the same HLA markers, only about a third of patients have a sibling with a matching HLA type. See the Blood and Marrow Transplant Information Network's website: http://www.bmtinfonet.org/before/beingrelateddonor, last accessed on October 15, 2016.

4. See the websites of the Organ Procurement and Transplantation Network and Transplant Living, respectively, at http://optn.transplant.hrsa.gov and www.trans plantliving.org, last accessed on October 15, 2016.

5. Ibid.

6. Ibid.

7. See the exposé by Kevin Sack, "Sixty Lives, Thirty Kidneys, All Linked," *New York Times,* February 18, 2012, http://www.nytimes.com/2012/02/19/health/lives -forever-linked-through-kidney-transplant-chain-124.html?_r=0. In fairness, paired exchanges are also associated with some interesting moral quandaries. First, kidney quality is never a constant. In cases with a single donor and a single recipient, this fact is simply a given. In paired exchanges it is more problematic: one donor may be better situated to donate a healthy kidney than the other. Also, in paired exchanges there is likely going to be unevenness in terms of where all parties get to choose the healthcare facilities they favor. How do decisions get made to preserve everyone's right to their preference of location for treatment? Finally, not all donor *pairs* are equal. Is it fair to ask a compatible pair to enter into a swapping arrangement with a less-compatible pair? For example, some blood types, for example, are rarer than others. Thanks to the anonymous reviewer for pointing out these complexities.

8. Ibid.

9. Ibid.

10. Ibid.

11. Ibid.

12. An example of one such company is Management Science Associates, whose product, EDIT, interfaces with UNOS data sets and is able to access labs, tissue typing, diagnostics, and other relevant features that determine biological and geographical suitability. EDIT puts to best use the mathematical algorithms that make paired exchanges and chains feasible in the first place. The company's website can be found here: http://msa.com/life-sciences/solutions/transplant-management-systems.

13. Danielle Ofri, "In Israel, a New Approach to Organ Donation," *New York Times*, February 16, 2012, http://well.blogs.nytimes.com/2012/02/16/in-israel-a-new-approach-to-organ-donation/?_r=0.

14. Ibid.

15. Ibid.

16. Ibid.

17. Dimitri Lindi, "Israel, a Leader in Transplant Tourism, Finds a Formula for Increasing Domestic Donations," *Tablet*, April 10, 2014, http://www.tabletmag.com/jewish-news-and-politics/164976/israel-organ-donation.

18. Richard Gray, "Registered Organ Donors Could Be Given Priority for Transplants," *Telegraph*, July 11, 2013, http://www.telegraph.co.uk/news/health/news/10172247/Registered-organ-donors-could-be-given-priority-for-transplants.html.

19. "Open Letter to President Barack Obama."

20. See the National Living Donor Assistance Program website: https://www.livingdonorassistance.org/Home/default.aspx, last accessed October 15, 2016.

21. Ibid.

22. Marilynn Marchione, "Wealth May Mean Health: Study Sees Advantage for Multiple Listing, Getting and Organ Transplant." *U.S. News,* November 9, 2015, http://www.usnews.com/news/us/articles/2015/11/09/wealth-may-give-advantage-for-getting-organ-transplants.

23. Ibid.

24. Givens, a transplant fellow at Columbia University Medical Center, found that higher death rates correlate with appearance on fewer listings. A comparison of people who appeared on one list versus on multiple ones: 12 percent versus 8 percent for those in search of a heart; 17 percent versus 12 percent for those in search of a liver; and 19 percent versus 11 percent for those in search of a kidney. See Raymond Givens, "The Wealthiest, Not the Sickest, Patients May Have the Edge in Organ Transplants," the abstract of which is accessible here: http://newsroom.heart.org/news/wealthiest-not-sickest-patients-may-have-edge-in-organ-transplants, last accessed October 15, 2016.

25. Givens found that only 12 percent of people seeking a kidney were able to afford multiple listings, making wealth not just a significant factor in terms of determining success but a relatively common one too.

26. Jon Stone, "Blood Donors in Sweden Get a Text Message Whenever Their Blood Saves Someone's Life," *Independent*, June 10, 2015, http://www.independent.co.uk/news/world/europe/blood-donors-in-sweden-get-a-text-message-whenever-someone-is-helped-with-their-blood-10310101.html.

27. Ibid.

28. As reported on the Johns Hopkins Medicine website: http://www.hopkinsmedicine.org/news/media/releases/the_facebook_effect_social_media_dramatically_boosts_organ_donor_registration, last accessed October 15, 2016.

29. See the UNOS website: https://www.unos.org/donation/honoring-donors/, last accessed October 15, 2016. For a complete list of names, see: https://www.unos.org/donation/honoring-donors/wall-of-names.

30. As reported on the website of LiveOnNY: http://www.liveonny.org/uploaded _files/tinymce/2016/Love_Life_Legacy_pamphlet.pdf, last accessed, October 15, 2016.

31. At the same time, big rewards in the form of funeral expenses, health insurance, or college tuition are arguably not that different than big financial payments and are perhaps even more morally problematic given their lack of transparency. By contrast, vouchers, or "promissory notes" on returned future kidneys, could easily be construed as a variant on paired exchanges and therefore not problematic in the same way. These issues beckon us to seriously consider how to interpret the prohibition in NOTA against exchanges for *valuable* consideration.

32. Enrique Rivero, "'Gift Certificate' Enables a Kidney Donation When Convenient and Transplant When Needed," *UCLA Newsroom*, July 11, 2016, http://news room.ucla.edu/releases/gift-certificate-enables-kidney-donation-when-convenient -and-transplant-when-needed.

33. Robert M. Veatch and Lainie F. Ross, *Transplantation Ethics*, 2nd ed. (Washington, DC: Georgetown University Press, 2015), 179.

34. See Martha C. Nussbaum, *The Fragility of Goodness: Luck and Ethics in Greek Tragedy and Philosophy* (Cambridge: Cambridge University Press, 1986).

35. Veatch and Ross, *Transplantation Ethics*, 181.

36. R. Schwindt and A. Vining, "Proposal for a Mutual Insurance Pool for Transplant Organs," *Journal of Health Politics, Policy and Law* 23 (1988): 725, 741, quoted in Veatch and Ross, *Transplantation Ethics*, 181.

37. Although, slowly, there are proposals on the state level to change this, such as in New York. See: http://www.crainsnewyork.com/article/20170223/HEALTH_CARE /170229960/albany-considers-bill-to-pay-live-organ-donors-costs.

Conclusion:
Two to Four Hours of Your Life

Save for a bad habit of sometimes failing to fasten my seatbelt when I'm driving, over the last several years I have enjoyed a strong driving record. At one point I shared with a friend the news of my occasional sin. She suggested that instead of spinning my wheels going to traffic court to try to talk my way out of minor violations of which I was obviously guilty, I should instead fight for a law that prevents a ticket if one can demonstrate that one has registered to become an organ donor. She had taken into account what I had told her about the long-run costs to society of providing dialysis versus facilitating kidney transplantations. Whatever the cost of individuals not wearing seatbelts who get in accidents and end up in operating rooms, this amount would be made up for and then some by the additional organs that would become available through such unorthodox incentives for becoming donors.

Her suggestion, proffered in a grinning, cynical fashion of someone who knew my flaws perhaps a tad more than I'd have preferred, was intended more as a prod for me to acquire better driving instincts than as perspicacious advice about the national organ donor situation. Nevertheless, my friend was also on to the kernel of truth reflected in many of the suggestions presented here: whatever we do as individuals should be done in a manner that has other-regarding implications. Public health policies make the biggest difference when they promote the idea that "we are all in this together." While my friend's idea won't solve the organ shortage problem by itself, it does highlight the sort of perspective-taking and outside-the-box thinking we need in order to get beyond the typical profit-driven incentives and individualism that hamper policy innovation in medicine today.

Unfortunately, the US system is often designed to do the opposite. In a medical culture marred by an emphasis on liability rather than the best interests of patients, policies are typically characterized by defensiveness over practicality. In terms of organ transplantation, the situation is no different. Dr. Adel Bozorgzadeh, a transplant surgeon at the University of Massachusetts Memorial Medical Center in Worcester, notes in a recent study that as a result of new guidelines regulating grafts, many US hospitals now dispose of any organs deemed to be less than perfect, thus withholding from some of their most ailing patients potentially lifesaving transplantations out of the concern that anything below optimal surgical outcomes will result in a federal investigation, crackdown, or even litigation.[1] Consequently, thousands of patients waiting for organs are not getting the assistance that could extend their lives, leading to a situation in which the "altruism of organ donation is being wasted."[2] Bozorgzadeh's study reviewed the cases of more than ninety thousand adult deceased donor liver transplant candidates at 102 transplant centers between 2002 and 2012; it links outcome-based auditing, in which transplant centers are penalized for reporting nonoptimal results, to the delisting of transplant candidates in desperate straits.[3] Delisting immediately increased by 16 percent at the time of the implementation of the new guidelines, and the likelihood of being delisted continued to increase by 3 percent per quarter thereafter.[4] The guidelines were intended to assure quality control, yet the new regulations ironically seemed to be leading to a situation in which fewer individuals are getting the help they needed. Instead of having a somewhat reduced chance of survival with a less-than-perfect organ, high-risk patients (the individuals normally eligible for these grafts) are given no chance at all. If an environment is created in which hospitals throw away donated organs in order to maintain high ratings, it is even more urgent to find ways to fight the inefficiencies that drag down a health system that is already too liability conscious and profit driven.

Since the writing of this book began, the transplantation waiting list has stabilized, but making this gain by delisting the sickest patients in our midst is not a desirable way to do it.[5] No doubt, it is always wise in medical ethics to bear in mind the conservative adage that just because we *can* do something doesn't mean we *should* do it. At the same time, adopting a too-cautious attitude about technological innovation needlessly deprives an immeasurably better life to victims of disease and trauma. Striking the right balance between technological optimism and ethical reservation is an art. In our changing world, the tendency to become more self-monitoring regulatorily and, as a result, more rule-conscious, should be balanced with availing ourselves of new options made possible by lifesaving and life-enhancing innovations that come through technology's ever-expanding frontiers.

Admittedly, such innovations inevitably thrust on our consciousness new ethical issues to consider. We must ask: What is equitable, safe, and worth promoting in a technology-reliant world? Arriving at moral clarity requires a process of ongoing mental recalibration. For example, should advances in biomedical engineering allow us artificially to replenish failing organs more reliably than we now do, the metric by which the need for costly sacrifice is assessed will undoubtedly have to change, as there will not be the same need for organ donors.[6] At present, however, we are still far from the day when the resource of willing human donors is anything short of precious and necessary.

Fortunately, medical defensiveness is not the only reason that the organ waiting list is beginning to stabilize. Surgical advances have made the transplantation process safer and more efficient on an ongoing basis, thus steadily making organ donation a less-drastic medical option than it has been for generations past. This fact, along with the serious effort to advertise transplantation safety and effectiveness now being exerted by organizations like UNOS and Donate Life, is likely responsible for the increase in transplantations occurring nationwide, a trend that certainly impacts the waiting list.[7] Between 2013 and 2014 the waiting list decline for all organs was 10 percent greater than each previous year, and it was an additional 6.5 percent between 2014 and 2015, with the same rate projected for 2015 and 2016.[8] This trend is specifically the result of fewer patients with failing livers needing transplantation due to new medications that are now available to individuals afflicted with hepatitis type C. (New antiviral therapy accounts for the 4,000 to 5,000 fewer patients listed by UNOS today.) This goes to show just how much technology can help the cause. Still, the overall number of those on the waiting list remains close to 120,000, and wait times for new organs persist. At Stony Brook Hospital the average listed patient's wait time for a kidney is at the moment between 1.14 years (for blood type AB) and 4.46 years (for blood type B).[9] This is, of course, longer than it should be. Furthermore, in this country the total cost of treating patients in kidney failure, the majority of whom are on dialysis, is nearly $35 billion. Obviously more needs to be done to recruit informed, willing donors.[10] The situation will become even more pressing in an era of expanding lifespans and fewer brain deaths, the natural result of which is to be able to depend less on cadaveric donation as medical advances continue to accumulate and which makes recruitment among a living donor population more important than ever.

Offering financial incentives to propel efforts in recruiting living donors will ultimately not be as effective as engendering a sense of civic engagement, regardless of what form that civic engagement takes. The question remains, however: What might inspire someone on an individual level and within the context of his or her own life to come to care about someone dying of kidney disease? In answering this question, one distinction made by the moral philosopher Shelly Kagan about the difference between "pale" and "vivid" beliefs comes to mind. Often we have an abstract, general sense about others who are suffering. But this concern remains purely academic and part of our generally accepted background set of beliefs that refer to what is wrong with the world. These pale beliefs, authentic and factually true as they may be, become vivid for us only when we acquire the conviction that urgently grips us in a way that morally interrupts the safety and routine of our everyday lives.

Kagan notes that we are most likely to care about the starving humans we see on late-night television infomercials once we also gain geographical proximity to them or develop some emotional connection that makes them more relatable than they were before, such as discovering that they share our ethnic or cultural background. It is not, Kagan points out, that the moral imperative to feed the impoverished was any less pressing before we came to care about them; pale and vivid beliefs share the same moral status. Rather, the "caring about" becomes the decisive part in terms of moral *action*.[11] Kagan's point is that once we realize that our pale beliefs are no less true than our vivid ones, we can begin to accept that our not having acted on them—which is often easier to do—was our own failing rather than because of any weakness of the veridical force of the beliefs themselves. As pale beliefs become more vivid, the urgency with which we dispose ourselves to help others expands as their situation simultaneously becomes a reality for us.

How might the generally pale (but true) belief that we ought to do what we can to help the plight of an individual waiting for an organ become a vivid one? My closing suggestion pertains to a minimal activity that could at most intrude faintly into our busy lives: devoting two to four hours of our lives to visit someone currently undergoing dialysis. This individual can be someone who is or is not personally known. The visit could take place at any dialysis center in the United States. The shared time could be facilitated by dialysis centers themselves, perhaps in pilot programs intended to bring together populations of people with healthy and dying kidneys. Such programs should ideally procure the consent of all involved parties. With little effort, space could be made to welcome visitors in the areas where patients receive dialysis. Programs would clearly entail no expectations beyond the introduction of two individuals. The goal is to guarantee an environment free of coercion. Two people would simply get to meet one another, get to know one another a little better, and, in this activity alone, learn something. With such learning experiences the "pale" familiarity with a noble cause becomes a vivid realization about the day-to-day existence of those for whom such a cause exists.

It is just these sorts of exposures to one another in life that will move mountains and save lives. It is safe to presume that many of these one-on-one encounters would end with nothing changing beyond the visitor perhaps making an appointment at the DMV to declare his or her status as an organ donor. However, some visitors might be moved to do something a little more. Whether that "more" amounts to "civic duty" or a sacrifice rendered "above and beyond" matters little. Certainly the label would not be significant when placed in the context of questions surrounding a new observable phenomenon. For example: What *would* the impact on society be if a dialysis center became known for facilitating the emergence of willing donors? As technology continues to advance, could donating a kidney become the "new" blood donation? As the risks of nephrectomy go down and the long-term success of a graft goes up, might "kidney donation campaigns" become a real thing? At the moment there is no way to know, but there is usually not a way to know the result of any important experiment at the experiment's outset.

This modest proposal—to simply think about how to create programs that make it easy for people to spend time with individuals on dialysis—will make money less relevant to solving the organ shortage problem, while community and collective action would become more relevant. This belief is founded on a faith in the nature of human beings: we are social beings who exist to act on opportunities to help one another provided we are supplied with a little help in seeing these opportunities come to fruition. But more than faith and benevolence will be required to get this experiment going in any real way. The idea presumes, minimally, that we will continue to get better at practicing medicine, and that the short- and especially long-term costs of undergoing a nephrectomy or the partial removal of a lobe of one's liver will gradually become less of a burden for the donor. We are not there yet, but the alternative—introducing price tags to induce kidney selling—assures that we will never get there.

It bears noting that the proposed experiment is the special kind for which failure is sometimes success at a further remove. Many donors reveal that the path they decided to follow was chosen because of a prior decision not to walk down a different one. We often do something today because of not having done something else yesterday. Individuals in kidney failure are not the only ones suffering on the planet, and there are endless repositories for our goodwill, but few of us, despite our best attempts to regulate our psychological constitution, will consider donating a kidney unless the recipient is someone who resides within our innermost circle. This is okay, for we will change ourselves, and the world, in some small way just by trying.

Herein lies one of the beautiful ironies involved in grand sacrifices like the one being considered: the gift that is rendered accrues great benefit to the giver, as much as the benefit that reaches the recipient. To say so is not simply charming idealism; it is a practical reality, witnessed and attested to by countless philanthropists, blood donors, volunteers of charitable organizations, first responders, rescuers of victims of genocide, and altruistic organ donors. It may be that nothing more than a little learning that occurs in a two-to-four-hour shift spent with someone whose daily reality is different than our own. This small act can still represent a shift from the "pale" to the "vivid." In this fact alone the limits of what is possible versus what isn't are redrawn, for ourselves individually and for society together.

NOTES

1. Casey Ross, "Hospitals Are Throwing Out Organs and Denying Transplants to Meet Federal Standards," *STAT*, August 11, 2016, https://www.statnews.com/2016/08/11/organ-transplant-federal-standards/.

2. Ibid.

3. Natasha H. Dolgin, Moyahedi Babak, Paulo N. A. Martins, Robert Goldberg, Kate L. Lapane, Frederick A. Anderson, and Adel Bozorgzadeh, "Decade-Long Trends in Liver Transplant Waitlist Removal Due to Illness Severity: The Impact of Centers for Medicare and Medicaid Services Policy," *Journal of the American College of Surgeons* 222, no. 6 (June 2016): 1054–65.

4. Ibid.

5. At its height at the end of 2014, close to 125,000 individuals were on the waiting list; as of the spring 2017 that number is just under 117,000. Indications are that this number will more likely rise again than fall further, and that the (in effect) one-time adjustment seems to have more to do with innovation with regard to combating hepatitis type C (and therefore with listings of patients waiting for a new liver) than anything else. Certainly the decrease by nearly 5,000 individuals is not significant in the context of the steady annual increases over the last twenty years. Other trends affecting the stabilization of the waiting list, such as the rise in the number of organs procured nationally due to tragic deaths caused by the opioid epidemic, are hopefully short-term.

6. Noting that their fruition is still ten or more years away, there are more than a few biomedically engineered organs on the horizon. For example, Johnson and Johnson's diabetes division, "Animas," has released word of a forthcoming artificial pancreas. See Andy Batts, "Johnson and Johnson's Artificial Pancreas May Be Launched Earlier Than Expected," *Seeking Alpha*, July 9, 2014, http://seekingalpha .com/article/2306345-johnson-and-johnsons-artificial-pancreas-may-be-launched -earlier-than-expected. Already new dialysis options exist for those suffering from renal disease. At the 2016 NATCO (Organization for Transplant Professionals) conference in Orlando, several booths featured the latest devices in home hemodialysis. One new product introduced by NxStage, for instance, called "System One," is a user-friendly, portable, and relatively small dialysis machine that allows individuals needing infusions to choose the time and place that is most convenient for them to undergo treatments. These options open up vistas for patients on dialysis, allowing them to maintain normal work schedules and travel easier. While these sorts of devices become better and more prevalent over time, the need for transplantation will, of course, become less pressing. But in terms of lifestyle and cost, transplantation will still be preferable. For more on NxStage's System One, see www.nxstage.com.

7. This is the view of Helen Irving, president and CEO of LiveOnNY, as discussed in an email exchange with her on September 8, 2016.

8. As interpreted by me from data retrieved from the following available website, which is overseen by the US government: https://optn.transplant.hrsa.gov/data/view -data-reports/build-advanced/, last accessed November 1, 2016.

9. These figures are based on internal data shared at monthly meetings of the Organ Donor Council at Stony Brook Hospital.

10. This figure, current through 2013, has continued to rise in the last three years. See the NIH factsheet: https://report.nih.gov/nihfactsheets/ViewFactSheet.aspx?csid =34, last accessed November 1, 2016.

11. Shelly Kagan, *The Limits of Morality* (Oxford: Oxford University Press, 1989), 283–91, 299–300, 304–7.

INDEX

abortion, 71
adoption, 91–92
Affordable Care Act, 29, 61
African Americans, 26
algorithms, 142–43, 157n12
allocation process, 25, 46, 48, 59
ALODN (American Living Organ Donor Network), 43
altruism: case studies of, 118; civic duty and, 106; coercion and, 38; domino effect and, 127–28; empathy and, 112–13, 122–24; financial compensation and, 5–6, 7, 58, 99; financial incentives and, 94, 111–12; health benefits of, 126–27; indirect compensation and, 102; as an intrinsic motivation, 81; Kravinsky and, 9–10, 21n21, 21n22; literature on, 15; profits and, 47; public acknowledgment and, 149; regulated market and, 47–48; removal of disincentives and, 138; self-interest and, 5, 6–7, 16–17, 74, 75, 76, 111; self-regard and, 17, 76, 106, 111, 112, 115, 132–33, 134, 152; stranger donors and, 21n21, 118, 121; unmotivated (pure), 111–14
Alvaro, Eusebio M., 15
American Living Organ Donor Network (ALODN), 43
Anjoman, 43–46, 48
anonymity, 8, 11–12, 21–22n25, 44, 101–2
The Antichrist (Nietzsche), 106
Aristotle, 74, 94, 113–14
artificial organs, 2–3, 17n10, 162, 166n6

Ashkenazi, Tamar, 145
attachment, formation of, 11
autonomy, 30, 32, 65, 132
awards, 90–91

bankable good programs, 151–52, 156
Barnhill, Anne, 107–8n19
Batson, C. Daniel, 112–13, 122
beliefs, pale vs. vivid, 163, 164, 165
Bender, Courtney, 12
Berger, Alexander, 29
best interests, 33, 41, 60, 63–64, 160–61
bioethics, 71, 79n45. *See also* ethical issues
biomedically engineered organs, 2–3, 17n10, 162, 166n6
black market, 41–42; alternatives to, 25, 53; in China, 64; exploitation and, 41, 52n38, 53; in India, 55; price of kidneys in, 77n4
blood donors, 8, 13, 59, 66, 78n36, 85–86, 148–49
blood supply, 4, 66–67, 78n36
bodies, stewardship of, 71
Bourdieu, Pierre, 76
Boyer, J. Randall, 63, 65
Bozorgzadeh, Adel, 161
brain death, 79n46, 144, 162
Bramstedt, Katrina A., 15, 122–24, 127
bribe effect, 90, 100
Broadman, Howard, 152
brokers, 41–42, 77n4
Brown, Michael, 126, 129
Brown, Stephanie, 126, 129

Feinberg, Joel, 31
financial compensation: altruism and, 5–6, 7, 58, 99; arguments for, 28–30; buy-in and, 87, 88, 95, 97, 98; contractual arrangements for, 38–39; equity and, 29–30; fairness and, 101–2; for financial hardships, 102, 146–48, 156; funds for, 25, 77n5; historical background of, 23–24; indirect forms of, 102; Iranian system and, 42–46, 52n48; literature on, 15; vs. lump-sum financial incentives, 99–102; motivation and, 9; vs. nonpayment, 5–6, 7; prohibition of, 139–40; reasonable, 147; removing disincentives and, 138; risks and, 84, 85; short- and long-term consequences of, 128
financial disincentives, 138, 139
financial incentives: altruism and, 94, 111–12; for blood, 66, 78n36; civic duty and, 10, 83, 88, 92–94, 99, 104, 107–8n19, 108n27, 108n28, 162–63; crowding-out thesis and, 13, 14, 85–86, 88, 94, 98, 107–8n19; donor-recipient relationship and, 101–2; economic disparity and, 96–98; for egg or sperm donation, 11, 29; as an extrinsic motivation, 81; vs. financial disincentives, 138; high priced, 89, 93, 108n28; historical background of, 23–24; impact of, 89, 156; lump-sum, 99–102, 112, 147, 151; for medical trials and experiments, 30; nuclear waste facility and, 87–89; psychological factors and, 82–83; public attitudes on, 96–98; rational actor theory and, 82; recruitment and, 85. *See also* commodification; monetization; organ market
fines, impact of, 93–94
Forgacs, Gabor, 19n10
Fox, Renée C., 14, 37
free choice, 32
freeloading, 95, 96
free market: beneficiaries of, 63; efficiency of, 40; exploitation and, 31; vs. gift exchanges, 12; proponents of, 5, 20n14; purpose of, 26–27; social relations and, 14; supply and demand problems in, 58. *See also* organ market

Free Market Institute, 20n14
Frey, Bruno: on the bribe effect, 90, 100; on collective goods, 151; on financial incentives, 13, 14; on nuclear waste facilities, 86–89; on trust, 95–96
Friedman, Amy: on the current situation, 1; on financial compensation, 30, 84–85; on legalization of organ sales, 39; on parents, 5, 130; on stranger donors, 17; on waiting with dignity, 7
friendship, 36, 90–91, 124
Frisch, Ragnar, 106n1
Fry-Revere, Sigrid, 15, 43–46, 52n48
fulfillment, 90, 92, 105, 132, 133, 134
fungible goods, 12–13, 72, 74, 92

Gandhi, 10, 21n22, 136n37
gender, paid surrogacy and, 34
"get-rich-quick" schemes, 63–64
gift exchange, 12, 13, 16, 76
gift giving, 11, 85, 102, 123–25, 165
The Gift Relationship (Titmuss), 13, 15
gifts: commodification of, 68, 70, 71–73, 76; definition of, 12; especially precious goods as, 39; freely offered, 10; as fungible goods, 12–13; organ donations defined as, 23, 24; purity of, 27; tyranny of, 37, 38
Gill, Jagbir, 97
Givens, Raymond, 148, 158n24, 158n25
giving act. *See* gift giving
Gneezy, Uri, 92–93, 108n27
goods: authentically rendered, 6, 7; bankable, 151–52, 156; collective nature of, 92, 151; commodification of, 13, 72, 89–98; comparable, 151–52, 159n31; contested, 68; demand for, 39; fungible, 12–13, 72, 74, 92; monetization of, 89–98; "sacred," 24; scarcity of, 25, 42; social, 8, 69, 100. *See also* especially precious goods
Good Samaritanship, 15, 124, 142
Goyal, Madhav, 62, 64
Grieving Wall, 150

Haidt, Jonathan, 127–28, 148, 152
Halachic Organ Donor Society (HODS), 49n3

prices and pricing: fixed, 46; high, 89,
108n28; of kidneys, 57, 77n4, 77n5;
regulated market for, 58
prisoners, Falun Gong, 55
procurement process, 24–25, 48, 49, 67, 73,
79–80n53
profits: alternatives to, 160; altruism and,
47; autonomy and, 30; black market,
41–42; for blood donors, 66, 78n36;
equity and, 35; ethical issues and, 55;
from health care services, 29, 50n12;
historical background of, 24; in Iran, 42;
by middlemen, 41–42, 62; self-interest
and, 70. *See also* financial incentives;
monetization
progesterone, 126
prosocial behavior, 113, 123, 128, 133
psychological factors: financial incentives
and, 82–83; in giving and receiving, 38,
39, 76, 85, 126–27; needy poor and,
63–64; paid surrogacy and, 34
public acknowledgment, 148–50
public awareness campaigns, 104–5
public health policy, 96, 160–61
public safety, 56, 64–68, 162
public spirit. *See* civic duty/engagement
pure (unmotivated) altruism, 111–14

quality of life, 124, 126
questionnaires, 67

Rabin, Yitzhak, 21n22
race, 83, 97
Radin, Margaret Jane, 33, 40, 68–69, 72
Randall, Peter, 41
rational actor theory, 82
receiving, act of, 85, 101, 133
recipients. *See* organ recipients
recruitment, 7, 47, 67, 82, 85, 104, 162
registered organ donors, 129, 145, 149, 156
regrets, 62, 64, 104, 126
regulated markets: in Iran, 42–46, 48,
52n48; myth of, 59; pricing in, 58;
public safety and, 67–68; role of, 24–25,
46–49; vs. unregulated, 31–32
Reid, Donnell, 9, 21n22
religions, 23, 24, 49n3, 56, 77n3, 79n46

rent seeking, 40
Richards, Janet Radcliffe, 5–6
Rodrigue, James, 104–5
Rosenbaum, Levy Izhak, 52n38
Ross, Lainie F., 15, 32–33
Rothman, David, 59
Rothman, Sheila, 59
Rousseau, Jean-Jacques, 94
Rustichini, Aldo, 92–93, 108n27
Ruzzamenti chain, 142–43

Sack, Kevin, 142–43
sacrifice. *See* self-sacrifice
sacrificial child, 57–58
sale of organs. *See* financial incentives;
legalization of organ sales; organ market
sanctity of life doctrine, 56, 70–71
Sandel, Michael, 69, 90–92, 93–94, 142
Satel, Sally, 1–2, 36–38, 140
Satz, Deborah, 61
scarcity, 25, 42. *See also* organ shortage
Schicktanz, Silke, 100–101
Schwindt, Richard, 154
Scientific Registry of Transplant Recipients
database, 148
self-esteem, 126
self-interest: altruism and, 5, 6–7, 16–17,
74, 75, 76, 111; bankable good programs
and, 152; vs. civic duty, 87; corrupting
nature of, 112; incentives and, 18;
Kravinsky and, 9; profits and, 70; virtue
and, 146
selfless behavior: elevation phenomenon
and, 128; empathy-altruism hypothesis
and, 112; evolutionary advantage of,
132; health benefits of, 126; motivation
and, 45, 145; organ market and, 76;
self-regard and, 6; virtues and, 113
self-regard, 111–14; altruism and, 17, 76, 106,
111, 112, 115, 132–33, 134, 152; donor
chains and, 143; financial incentives
and, 82; Israeli program and, 144–45;
motivation and, 6, 122, 151–52, 154;
other-regard and, 45; selfless behavior
and, 6; self-sacrifice and, 14
self-sacrifice: altruism and, 15, 111, 113,
124; benefits of, 165; civic duty

ABOUT THE AUTHOR

Andrew Michael Flescher is a member of the Core Faculty, Program in Public Health; professor of Family, Population, and Preventive Medicine; and professor of English at the State University of New York, Stony Brook. A member of the United Network for Organ Sharing Ethics Committee, he is the author of several books, including *Moral Evil* and *Heroes, Saints, and Ordinary Morality*, both from Georgetown University Press.

CPSIA information can be obtained
at www.ICGtesting.com
Printed in the USA
LVOW08*1740210318
570657LV00008B/197/P